ADDITION/
THE MENOPAUSE м т ...

"Reading Dr. Arianna's book, *The Menopause Myth*, was like having a conversation with a really good friend who cares enough to listen to you and roll up her sleeves to help you. This book will change the game by starting a conversation about women's health that liberates, educates, and gets us really excited about 'the change.' I'm ready!"

—Leslie Fuqua Williams, coach and host of GatherAndShine

"Finally, honest talk about an important transition in life that affects women and everyone in their worlds. This book will save your sanity and relationships."

—Kate Delaney, Emmy award-winning nationally syndicated talk show host and author of *Deal Your Own Destiny*

"Dr. Arianna has pulled it off yet again! In *The Menopause Myth: What Your Mother, Doctor, and Friends Haven't Told You about Life after 35*, she gets to the heart of the matter by articulating what no one else has about a very sensitive and personal topic for myself and many other women—the midlife change, a.k.a. menopause. For me, she has been an angel at two pivotal moments in my life: during the pregnancy and birth of my premature son and now during my midlife 'transition.' Dr. A's wisdom, intellect, and integrative approach to health and wellness are lifesavers and have helped me and my husband better understand and navigate the mysterious things that are happening in my body and impact so much of what I do. *The Menopause Myth* is a must-read for women of all ages but especially those who might feel that they are not themselves and want to understand what may be occurring as they approach their forties. In this book, Dr. A first describes her own journey through menopause and then utilizes her clinical expertise to discuss and debunk myths associated with menopause. There are real examples and meaningful solutions included to help women bring balance back to their lives and excel during their journey through menopause!"

—Charlotte Jones-Burton, MD, MS,
president and founder of Women of Color in Pharma

THE
MENOPAUSE
MYTH

ARIANNA SHOLES-DOUGLAS, MD

THE MENOPAUSE MYTH

WHAT YOUR *MOTHER*, *DOCTOR*, AND *FRIENDS*
HAVEN'T SHARED ABOUT *LIFE AFTER 35*

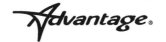

Published by Advantage, Charleston, South Carolina.
Member of Advantage Media Group.

ADVANTAGE is a registered trademark, and the Advantage colophon is a trademark of Advantage Media Group, Inc.

Printed in the United States of America.

10 9 8 7 6 5 4 3 2 1

ISBN: 978-1-59932-894-2
LCCN: 2019911286

Cover design by Jamie Wise.
Interior design by Carly Blake.

This publication is designed to provide accurate and authoritative information in regard to the subject matter covered. It is sold with the understanding that the publisher is not engaged in rendering legal, accounting, or other professional services. If legal advice or other expert assistance is required, the services of a competent professional person should be sought.

 Advantage Media Group is proud to be a part of the Tree Neutral® program. Tree Neutral offsets the number of trees consumed in the production and printing of this book by taking proactive steps such as planting trees in direct proportion to the number of trees used to print books. To learn more about Tree Neutral, please visit **www.treeneutral.com**.

Advantage Media Group is a publisher of business, self-improvement, and professional development books and online learning. We help entrepreneurs, business leaders, and professionals share their Stories, Passion, and Knowledge to help others Learn & Grow. Do you have a manuscript or book idea that you would like us to consider for publishing? Please visit **advantagefamily.com** or call **1.866.775.1696**.

To my patients, who teach me daily.

CONTENTS

FOREWORD

And just like that, the entire room gasped! A presentation slide with fifteen vaginas appeared and the entire room of ladies attending Dr. Arianna's talk covered our faces, blushed, and felt immediately uncomfortable as if we thought she was going to call it a "thingy" and not really give us the grown woman talk; after all, the presentation was about our lady parts.

That was the first day I met Dr. Arianna. She was doing an event in her office called "What's going on down there?" I stumbled across this on social media as I looked for things to do in my new town, Tucson, AZ. I had only been in Tucson a week and when I saw this beautiful, black female gynecologist having an event with wine and food, I signed up. She has always been humbled as to how I found her that day. I guess she had no idea she was actually quite famous in this desert town. And she was my first friend.

After that day, I have often wondered why women are curious but scared to really know about our vaginas. Who taught us that it was okay to be freaky with the lights off but scared to actually see the life-giving, pleasure-seeking, pink, warm, juicy vagina? Throughout the time I've known Dr. Arianna, I've seen this presentation a few times, and I am still shocked every time she puts up that slide and I watch a room full of women shrink. I told her that her message is so necessary and that we all need her to help us grow up. It's time we come out of this era of ignorance about our bodies, and we need her to guide us on this journey.

It really makes you wonder why we are not willing to address the elephant in the room. I mean, after all, women create life, shape future generations, bestow wisdom upon a nation, and extend grace to humanity in exchange for what?

How is it okay that women are riddled in confusion, tossed aside to make do, and cast away as what used to be a beautiful, young, juicy girl when it comes to our aging bodies?

To be empowered by the knowledge imparted in this book changes the game. Not only am I proud to be a woman because we are the most awesome creators ever, but I also know that getting older is a superpower. Dr. A gives power to us ladies, connecting dots to the most ignored medical myth that has kept us from truly living our best lives. Well the cat is out of the bag! As Dr. A says, menopause is "the journey to becoming who we were meant to be." Let's not dread the day but be empowered to participate in this event that is an "opportunity to reinvent or recreate yourself and become a stronger more authentic version of ourselves."

So, ladies, put on your yoga pants and grab a smoothie minus the sugar and acknowledge how brilliant God is for creating a woman— "the dress rehearsal is over, and your real life is right in front of you waiting to be embraced."

Oh, and don't be shy, Dr. A will put it all on the table. So be warned, and get a good mirror so you can see for yourself "what's going on down there."

Dr. A, this is right on time. Thank you!

— **Leslie Fuqua Williams**, *coach, speaker, and host of GatherAndShine—connecting women to what they truly desire*

THE "M" WORD

I was recently speaking with a friend who had just turned forty about the upcoming release of my book. She responded, "I can't wait to read it, but I'm not there yet." I chuckled at first, knowing that this book was written *exactly* for her and the countless women like her who think the menopause conversation does not pertain to them. Then I shared something that took her by surprise: a menopause myth.

I explained that one of the most widely held myths about menopause is that menopause doesn't affect women until *after* menstrual cessation. In other words: the myth is that your period disappears before you experience any menopause-like symptoms. The reality? Perimenopause—one of the most emotionally and hormonally tumultuous times of a woman's life—*precedes* menopause and starts as early as age thirty-five.

By age forty, you can almost be certain that you have begun *the journey*. This journey is not only heralded by the fluctuations of hormones, but also by a "personal awakening" that starts to occur.

Research professor and acclaimed author Brené Brown describes this period aptly: "Midlife is not a crisis. Midlife is an unraveling."[1] I could not agree more.

Awakening and unraveling. Midlife and menopause. It's all part of the journey that we'll talk about in this book.

My journey began without me being aware of it at first, when I had two young children, a husband, and the responsibilities of directing the High-Risk Pregnancy Center at Mercy Hospital in Baltimore, Maryland. Little did I know, I was stepping right into the middle of my midlife merry-go-round.

By age thirty-nine, I had checked all of the life boxes: college, medical school, residency, maternal fetal medicine fellowship, high-paying job, marriage, two kids, and nice house and car to boot. Despite all of these accomplishments, I felt empty, flat, anxious, and uninspired. I noticed visible signs of aging. I began reassessing my life's meaning and goals. I asked a lot of questions.

What had I accomplished? Was I on the trajectory I had set? What did that even mean? Why was I an irritable, hot mess? Why did I feel like my body, and especially my mind, were starting to betray me?

Throw in some fluctuating hormones, and finding the answers to my questions became quite tricky. I became exhausted, petulant, and devoid of libido. Ultimately, I was out of touch with my body and confused about all of the emotions that were surfacing.

But at that point in my journey, none of my experiences pointed to what I understood as menopause. Menopause was for "women over fifty with hot flashes, who are drying up, and living sexless lives marking the beginning of the end," a characterization I've heard hundreds of times. Sounds harsh, right?

---

1   Brené Brown, "The Midlife Unraveling," On Midlife, May 24, 2018, https://brenebrown.com/blog/2018/05/24/the-midlife-unraveling/.

No wonder women have traditionally avoided the "M" word like the plague. Who would want to talk or think about a life like that? How is it that a word that describes a period that lasts for almost a third of a woman's life is spoken in whispers, if spoken at all? This avoidance of information, resources, and conversations does a disservice to women and their families. It's not a myth; it's a reality. *Menopause* is not a dirty word. It's time we use it, reform it, and own it.

MYTH

Menopause is the beginning of the end.

REALITY

Menopause is a journey toward your best,
most authentic self.

Everyone knows that teenagers are hormonal. We expect the mood swings and other confusing behaviors. Likewise, we all know that pregnant women can be impacted by hormonal fluctuations. For pregnancy, there are classes, tours, books, TV shows, and professionals available to help the first-time mother. But for hormonal life after age thirty-five, the resources are unclear, less available, or filled with myths that offer us little practical knowledge.

So by age forty, I had no idea that I was already well into perimenopause. Furthermore, beyond the medical definition of *perimenopause*, I had no clue that I was a walking poster child with all of the symptoms. Even as an obstetrician/gynecologist with fifteen years of experience practicing medicine, I was clueless. How was that even possible? All I had learned in medical school and residency was that perimenopause precedes menopause. There were no conversations about what that really meant for a woman, not to mention the friends and family who had to deal with her.

Years passed before I recognized what was happening with me. The collision of midlife awakening and hormonal shifts continued to be ugly and unpleasant. As I eventually learned, the menopausal journey is not just about fluctuating hormones; it's about the convergence of midlife angst with hormonal upheaval. The journey is ultimately about balancing the emotional, physical, and spiritual components of coming into our own. Sound easy? It's not.

> The journey is ultimately about balancing the emotional, physical, and spiritual components of coming into our own.

MYTHS AND MENOPAUSE

Much of what we think we know about menopause is a myth. Perhaps the most prevalent myth is that menopausal symptoms are strictly physical. The fact is, our hormones also go on a journey, which leads to symptoms that aren't physical. When these occur, many women at midlife start to doubt their own sanity and stability. It's true that menopause can lead to some of the stereotypical symptoms we've all heard about, but as you will learn in this book, there are many more factors involved in the menopause journey. Recognizing the signs early can mean the difference between years of suffering and confusion versus years of living and understanding.

How did the menopause myths begin? The reasons are too many to count, but let's start with the obvious—and blame your mother. (Why not? Everyone else blames the mother!) In interviewing patients about how and where they receive their information about menopause, they rarely mention their mothers. The same mothers who made your period cake, doted over your first pregnancy, or helped you manage the first few days of motherhood have remained silent on the issue of menopause. Why? Because mothers, like most teachers, are incapable of imparting knowledge that they don't have. Furthermore, if your friends are unaware about their own bodies and journeys through menopause, they can't offer you any advice either. In fact, many circles of friends are all feeling the same things, with no clear teacher in sight.

It gets worse. Not only are your mother and friends mostly unprepared to help you navigate this period, but your doctor may be just as unprepared to help. The ignorance surrounding this phase of life is astounding when you consider that, on average, it lasts a decade and has life-changing impacts on quality of life, relationships, and work. Women are blindly struggling, with no viable solutions offered by their medical providers. If you have found a provider who takes the time to educate you and do more than simply prescribe a hormone or antidepressant, then you're fortunate.

Although there are many healthcare providers in front of the curve helping patients manage this phase, there are just as many, if not more, who do not possess the tools to help and who infuse their own misperceptions into their guidance. In addition, there is no consensus on the role of hormone replacement in women. Just within the past two decades, the pendulum has swung from offering hormones like candy to withholding hormones from desperate women entering menopause.

Are you confused yet? You're not alone. For years, I've been asking women what's the first thing that comes to mind when they hear the word *menopause*. I get a variety of answers and they usually involve metaphors of things sagging, shriveling, or drying up. *Menopause* sounds like a boogeyman who has come to rob us of our youth, vitality, and sexuality. It's surprising we don't have nightmares about it.

My next question: "Has anyone—a mother, aunt, any female figure—ever sat down and talked to you about menopause?" The answer is almost always no. How can it be that as grown women entering this stage of life, we are so woefully unprepared? Especially nowadays when, as the population ages, lifespans are longer and the average woman lives one-third of her life after menopause. Then I ask: "How comfortable or prepared do you feel entering peri/menopause?" I usually get a wide-eyed expression and a mumbled, "I don't really know."

I use the common menopause analogy of the grape versus the raisin; I explain that estrogen is a hormone that keeps everything juicy. As we age and estrogen levels fall, that juicy grape looks and feels more like a raisin. When I start speaking about the different symptoms of menopause, like vaginal dryness, painful intercourse, and decreased libido, most women over thirty-five nod—"Yes, I'm experiencing that!" Often, women don't correlate those symptoms with being perimenopausal.

In a recent Facebook poll, I asked women what their perceptions were of menopause. Several of the answers were expected and many of them were hilarious. It was obvious to me that the women who were informed about the role diet, exercise, and emotional work play in menopause seemed to have a much easier time.

"Menopause sucked. I know HRT [Hormone Replacement Therapy] is frowned upon, but it saved me from going stark-raving mad. For me, the first part was nearly nonstop hot flashes." —P.S.

"I'm pretty sure I'm going to spontaneously combust! And, uh, the mood swings... And sex?? I remember sex..." —D.B.

"Menopause is great! No periods, no birth control, can go swimming anytime! Less worries about stupid stuff. With plant-based nutrition and lots of exercise, no symptoms and lots of energy. Best times." —J.S.

Menopause is not a health emergency. It might feel like one when you are uneducated and unprepared, but it is a normal part of womanhood. In starting a conversation on menopause, my goal is to educate women about their physical changes and offer new technologies and remedies that alleviate the suffering of menopause.

The purpose of this book is to help you begin to wrap your head around the beautiful and equally frustrating experience, especially as a result of hormonal changes. Though I have not encompassed every aspect of aging, I have tried to address many of the myths that countless patients have approached me about. As you will discover, your lifestyle, specifically the food you put in your mouth, the company you keep, your thoughts, and especially your willingness to embrace "the change" are keys.

MY BACKGROUND IN INTEGRATIVE MEDICINE

I went into medicine because of one woman who showed me that doctors can change lives. She was my personal doctor, and she showed me firsthand how changing the quality of someone's life is the best gift that you can give. As a teenager, I had severe PMS with debilitating cramps. I was a cheerleader, on the track team, and was a pretty social kid. All things came to a standstill, however, when my cycle started. The pain was excruciating, and I would vomit for hours. I could only put a bucket at my bedside and pray that this month wouldn't be as bad as the last. Knowing that I could not tolerate this monthly ordeal for decades, I even contemplated suicide. Family and friends thought my condition was "mental." My mother took me to a few medical providers (pediatricians, therapists) who had nothing to offer. She eventually took me to a gynecologist who instantly diagnosed me and treated me with the equivalent of ibuprofen. My life changed overnight. I was able to engage in all of my activities almost without a hitch. I knew at that point that I wanted to change lives just as that gynecologist had affected mine.

I went into medicine with a sense of wonder and a mission to change the world. Of course, with a goal that lofty, it didn't quite happen that way. I started as a resident bursting with excitement and knowledge. The thrill quickly faded with the standard resident hazing, long nights on call, thousands of deliveries, and countless patients needing more than I had to give some days. In the last several years of practicing maternal-fetal medicine, I struggled in part because there was not a lot of space and time for patients to make major lifestyle changes while going through a complicated pregnancy. I realized that there was no real opportunity for me to establish long-term relationships and help women make life changes. Not knowing how it would change my life, I completed a fellowship in integrative medicine at the University of Arizona, founded by Dr. Andy Weil. One year later, with blissful ignorance, I opened an integrative wellness practice, Tula Wellness and Aesthetics.

As my practice grew, so did its scope. We added aesthetics services, as women continued to request technologies that could help them manage the physical changes they were seeing. I have to admit that I was reluctant to enter the aesthetics world. Over the years, however, it's become apparent that what a woman sees when she looks in the mirror is directly related to how she feels and takes care of herself. I realized that a woman's health starts with her aesthetic concerns and that self-perception plays an integral role in systemic health.

My approach to menopause and healthcare might be incongruent with what you have been taught. I have been trained to treat patients through the conventional lens of medicine, but over the years I have realized that there is nothing conventional about me. I have always wanted to treat patients with a more holistic approach. But on more than a few occasions, I was considered the "oddball," talking about how stress and diet affect a patient's health. It wasn't until the first day of my integrative medicine fellowship that I realized that there was an entire community of physicians who thought similarly. Mentorship from thought leaders and physicians such as Dr. Andy Weil gave me the courage to step out of traditional medicine and start a practice dedicated to integrative women's health.

MY JOURNEY FROM MENOPAUSE MYTH TO REALITY

I should say that don't like the term *menopause*. Defining women through the prism of their hormonal experience is a bad place to start, but since we must start somewhere, I'll start with my own journey.

In my late thirties, I started experiencing night sweats and worsening PMS. I was still menstruating regularly, so it never occurred to me that I was starting to experience perimenopause. By age forty-two, I found that I was irritable more often than not. As much as I loved my family, I felt disgusted and annoyed by every human being in the house. Driving home, I would pray that everyone was out running errands and that I would have the house to myself. It's true that we all get irritated with our partners sometimes, and often those annoyances are warranted, but I began to notice that my frustrations were escalating even without provocation.

One day I came home to find a dark kitchen. I could hear my husband, who hadn't noticed I had come home, watching football in the den. I was hungry and tired from a long day's work. That morning, I had asked my family to take out a semi-prepared meal and get dinner started, but apparently my message was not clear. Someone had taken the ingredients out of the fridge, and that was it. Nothing was even removed from the wrappings, much less chopped and ready to cook. Enough! I grabbed my keys, walked out the door, and went to a restaurant up the road to have dinner alone. When I returned home, my hungry family looked confused. My husband asked, "Did you come home earlier?" I said smugly, "Yeah, I did." I poured a glass of wine and retired to my room.

Things continued to worsen. I would look at my husband with disdain. In fact, I started having homicidal thoughts. I literally Googled "ways to poison your spouse." (However, I had watched enough *Dateline* and *20/20* shows to know that I'd already implicated myself by doing an internet search.) Yep, I went there. I told you it was bad.

My constant irritability coupled with bouts of brain fog contributed to a smoldering depression that was ready to create havoc on the rest of my life. The brain fog was so intense that, at one point, I was certain that I was suffering from early Alzheimer's. In fact, one day while performing a routine C-section, like the thousands I had performed before, my brain completely froze. I could not remember what the next step was to a procedure I normally could perform with my eyes closed. I remember thinking this was surely the beginning of the end for my career. Luckily, I was with a great surgical assistant who moved so fast I didn't have to worry about finishing the case. But it left me feeling confused and helpless.

My symptoms continued to become more pronounced. When I

finally connected the dots, I was embarrassed. The truth is, I missed my own diagnosis! Even as a female doctor of women's health, it took me five years to realize that my thought disturbances were symptoms of perimenopause. It was a dark and scary time that finally got better after dealing with all of the hormonal changes, adjusting my lifestyle, and sending out lots of prayers.

Despite my struggles, I make no apologies for my journey or for the work required to get to this place. It was not always a happy place; in fact, some days were downright miserable. I thought that being equipped with sixteen years of school and training and twenty years of medical practice would prepare me for the changes to come. I was wrong. Despite all my training, I was unprepared.

MYTH

Gynecologist are trained and prepared to discuss menopause and sexual health with patients.

REALITY

Conventional gynecological medical training focuses on reproductive health for women. Other specialties include high-risk pregnancy management, gynecological oncology, reproductive endocrinology, and urogynecology. Medical students and residents receive minimal training on mental, physical, and spiritual aspects of women's health after age forty.

I received extensive formal instruction in women's health, and yet I didn't learn about perimenopause in medical school, nor did I deal with it in residency. I remember a lot of conversations about pregnancy, and that my rotations were centered around labor and delivery, office gynecology, and gynecologic surgery. Most of the training revolved around a woman's reproductive phase. We had courses or rotations where we dealt with endocrinology, or the study of hormones, but everything was geared toward reproductive endocrinology (infertility) with little conversation about a woman's second half of life. Where women spend the most time, conventional medicine spends the least, and so it's become the phase where we lack the most understanding.

After twenty years of practicing maternal-fetal medicine, I retired from managing high-risk pregnancies and started my practice, Tula Wellness and Aesthetics. I now specialize in women's integrative health and functional medicine. I listen to the intimate details of women's lives on a daily basis. When I first started my practice in 2013, I began noticing a pattern in my patients' feedback that correlated with my own experience. I actually found some solace in hearing other women in similar predicaments. I realized that though the homicidal thoughts weren't healthy or functional, the extreme irritability, weight gain, fuzzy thinking, and hair loss I was concurrently experiencing were symptoms my patients were also citing. I was hearing the same thing day after day after day. Knowing that I wasn't "crazy" and that it wasn't "all in my head" was a powerful, transformative realization that completely changed my relationship with this phase of my life. I realized that I can start this conversation with other women. I can give them the same validation that proved so beneficial in my own journey.

You're Not Alone, and You're Not Crazy

When I was experiencing my own "mysterious" symptoms, some of which made me nearly homicidal, I did not understand there was a pattern to my symptoms or ways that I could alleviate them. I thought I was losing my edge, my sanity. The most important guidance I can initially offer women older than thirty-five is that you are not alone, and you are not crazy. You are experiencing the normal, biological progression of life. These hormonal fluctuations can have you feeling like you're sliding down a slippery slope without a recovery rope.

Embrace the Change

So many women view this time of life with complete confusion and a sense of dread. They start to focus on the signs of aging that we *all* experience. Hair loss, spare tires around the middle, and sagging faces are not-so-subtle reminders that we are indeed changing. There is technology available to push back the hands of time, and we will discuss them in later chapters, but the real work is mental and spiritual. At midlife, we are forced to take inventory of our lives and the decisions we've made to get us to this point. Unfortunately, we are not always happy with those decisions and where we are. This is where the work starts. Being honest with yourself is sometimes unpleasant, and you may find there are regrets, lingering resentment, and almost always some dreams deferred.

Do You!

Without proper insight, many symptoms of menopause can throw you for a loop and leave you wondering, "Who am I?" "What am I here to do?" In fact, it's not just menopause that creates this mindset. With an average life expectancy of eighty-one years, by the time you are in your mid-forties, it's safe to assume you have lived more years that you have left. So what are you waiting for? It's time to do you. Your life is waiting for you to show up, which always takes courage and sometimes means making some hard decisions.

THE MENOPAUSE CONVERSATION YOU SHOULD BE HAVING WITH YOUR DOCTOR

Forty years ago, nobody really recognized perimenopause as a significant issue worthy of understanding, much less of research and conversation. Women just dealt with it and suffered in silence. The women brave enough to mention these subtle changes to their doctors received little information. Unfortunately, the current healthcare model still doesn't allow time for doctors to truly assess a woman's physical and emotional symptoms.

> The current healthcare model still doesn't allow time for doctors to truly assess a woman's physical and emotional symptoms.

Today, traditional gynecologists survive in the healthcare system by either having a high volume of patients or by doing procedures. Procedures are typically reimbursed by insurance at a much higher rate than is time spent educating. The subtleties of guiding women through this phase require time spent talking and educating the patient. It's not something you can accomplish in a typical fifteen-minute visit. If you subtract the time spent on pleasantries and Pap smears, there's not a lot of time to devote to a woman's holistic health.

In addition to not having the time to discuss these important issues, there are, unfortunately, many personal biases that physicians project onto patients. I continue to be astounded by the ignorance surrounding menopause in the medical field. My patients often tell me things like: "My doctor said she doesn't believe in hormones," or, "My doctor told me I can't possibly be going through menopause because I'm too young." Most recently, a patient confided in me that her gynecologist of fifteen years told her it was *normal* to have pain with intercourse, after all, she had been with her husband twenty-five years. Therefore, she could not (and should not) expect to enjoy sex all of the time. That was perhaps the most depressing thing I had ever heard.

For these reasons, at Tula Wellness and Aesthetics, the first visit with all patients is somewhere between forty-five minutes to an hour. We discuss diet, stressors, and even what brings joy. Doctors and patients need to have real conversations about what this life-changing phase is all about. Many gynecologists don't take the adequate time to educate women about the five to ten years preceding menopause, or even entirely recognize perimenopause as one the most significant and life-changing experiences of a woman's life.

What has made me an advocate and menopause revolutionist is my own disillusionment and frustration with the system—doctors aren't trained to help women and many don't understand all of the factors that affect the symptoms of menopause. Unfortunately, patients are sometimes ignored or given inaccurate information. Some providers pretend like the ephemeral "M" word just doesn't exist. This is harmful to women's bodies and their psyches. I have heard countless scenarios where women were completely dismissed or placed on antidepressants for normal menopausal symptoms. No wonder women have kept silent about the changes in their bodies and minds.

But times are changing. There's still a significant amount of ignorance, fear, and misunderstanding, but women are evolving and are more apt to ask the questions. Today, the average American woman's lifespan is eighty-one years;[2] that means she's going to start experiencing perimenopause between ages thirty-five to forty-five, if not earlier. A woman spends most of her life—what is often consid-

---

2   "Average Life Expectancy in North America for Those Born in 2018, by Gender and Region (in Years)," Statista, accessed May 1, 2019, https://www.statista.com/statistics/274513/life-expectancy-in-north-america/.

ered the prime of her life, no less—dealing with some pretty intense hormonal changes. How is it that we can spend this much time in this hormonal phase, and yet women and the medical community remain so uninformed? Women are prepared for puberty and pregnancy but not for anything beyond. I always think of the maiden/mother/crone archetypes. Once you're no longer maiden or child bearing, all that remains is crone. Yikes! No wonder we all expect to dread this phase of life. The best way to mitigate fear and find a place of power, however, is through knowledge.

Fortunately, there is a new generation of women who demand understanding and validation of their bodies and their sexuality after midlife.

I want women and the medical providers who care for them to pay attention to how their bodies are changing. I want to empower women who feel like their providers turn a deaf ear to their complaints. I hope to start the real menopause conversation, open it up wide, so that it is destigmatized, demystified, and accessible to all women, their partners, their daughters, and mothers. It's an exciting time because there are new therapies and options available so women can continue to lead vital, pleasurable, fulfilled lives.

> I hope to start the real menopause conversation, open it up wide, so that it is destigmatized, demystified, and accessible to all women, their partners, their daughters, and mothers.

Part of the mission of this book is to give women the tools they need to understand how their bodies are changing. The most powerful tool is understanding. Integrating science and holistic health has become the trademark of my practice and my mission. By understanding that your body is always changing and that there are ways you can control how you're feeling, you keep your power. The revolutionary part of menopause, and what I try to instill in all of my patients, is that embracing it and understanding it can have truly transformative effects in women's lives.

Rather than be silent about it, and speak in hushed, fearful tones about the "M" word among our closest peers, let's talk brazenly about menopause. Embrace it. Let's converse about our sexual pleasure, our vaginal sensations, our thoughts and emotions, and let's demand that our doctors hear us and respond to us. This is how you can dispel the menopause myth and reclaim your life.

HOW TO READ THE MENOPAUSE MYTH

This book is not a memoir or a textbook about menopause; after all, there are plenty of those to reference. You won't find here a Band-Aid solution to speed through the discomfort, because one doesn't exist. But if you're interested in understanding how to ride this midlife rollercoaster, then reading this book is a good start. You'll learn how the mind, body, and spirit play roles in helping you transition into the best half of your life. The book has three sections:

- In chapters 1–5, we will debunk the most common menopause myths and delve into the science of the hormones that are most frequently out of balance.

- In chapters 6–7, we will look at how food, inflammation, and the gut all factor into peri/menopause.

- Finally, in chapter 8, we will explore the mental and spiritual aspects of self-care, and examine the "Jewels for the Journey."

***

Writing this book has not been easy and there have been countless distractions to pull me away from the work. Creating a roadmap through menopause for readers forced me to look even more closely at my own journey. The mental, physical, and spiritual work that is required to meet our highest selves, is always present—sometimes daunting and never finished. But in entering the second half of life, there is a silent acknowledgment that you better get it together. The dress rehearsal is over, and your real life is right in front of you, waiting to be embraced. Though there are frustrations along the way, infinite opportunities await.

Considering I was an ob-gyn who missed her own perimenopause diagnosis, I realized that peri/menopause is undoubtedly one of the most unrecognized and misunderstood times of a woman's life. This gap in information and resources compelled me to write this book.

If I could offer women a better understanding of this period in their lives, and offer frank discussions about the "M" word that so many people are afraid to discuss, then I might alleviate the confusion and suffering of many women in their midlives and beyond. My hope is that the guidance found in these pages will help to validate women and empower them to embrace a period of their lives that holds great power and wisdom.

CHAPTER 1

DISPELLING THE MENOPAUSE MYTHS

Tonya was a fifty-year-old patient who arrived at my clinic at the recommendation of her psychiatrist. She was a high-functioning woman who worked as an engineer, but she had recently found it difficult to keep up with the rigors of her daily life. She first consulted with her primary care doctor with symptoms of profuse night sweats and crippling anxiety—issues she had never experienced in the past. Her doctor sent her to a psychiatrist, who started her on two antidepressants, an antianxiety medication, and a sleeping pill. She had been on these medications for four months and had minimal relief in her symptoms. Thankfully, the psychiatrist (despite mistreating her with antidepressants and sleeping pills) suspected that these symptoms might be hormonally related to menopause.

In my office, Tonya described her symptoms to me, which were classic menopausal symptoms. I was frustrated that a medical professional such as the woman's psychiatrist could be so ignorant about common conditions affecting menopausal women. I placed Tonya on a Food Elimination Diet (which we will discuss in chapter 6) and, eventually, hormone replacement therapy (HRT). Under my care, she experienced relief from almost all of her symptoms and was able to sleep through the night. Eventually, I was also able to wean her off of the antidepressants and sleeping pills.

This is the experience of thousands of women who have been placed on antidepressants instead of dealing with the root cause of their symptoms—hormone imbalance. I'm certainly not suggesting that every woman with symptoms needs to be on hormones. In Tonya's case, as is the case for most of my patients, once we managed her relationship with food and begin some supportive supplements, there was a drastic reduction in symptoms.

Menopause is the beginning of our journey to become who we are meant to be.

As we will see in this chapter, one of the major myths of menopause is that it only relates to the menstrual cycle, or the end of it. In actuality, menopause is the beginning of our journey to become who we are meant to be. Menopause is about finding the courage and strength to be our authentic selves. Though there are physical changes in our hormones and bodies, there are emotional and spiritual changes that can help guide us toward our life's purpose. We just need to be aware of them and have the courage to pursue them.

THE MENOPAUSE IS COMING!
THE MENOPAUSE IS COMING!

Every woman knows that "the menopause is coming," but no one knows exactly when it will happen or what state they will be in once it's over. Even if we consider ourselves educated, well-informed consumers of medical care, we're still not convinced that we have this one in the bag.

At worst, we are overtaken by symptoms and ignorance of the process and lose ourselves; at best, we enter menopause with a nervous confidence that we will survive this just as we have survived every other stage of life. After all, we are women, we are resilient, we got this! Right?

Perhaps this is why our foremothers didn't have this conversation with their daughters, sisters, or friends. Perhaps this is why doctors have traditionally done little to inform patients about this time in their lives. Maybe they knew the truth about women—with everything we carry on our shoulders, the journey through menopause is just another reality that we will manage.

Regardless of the reasons, the conversations haven't happened. The chasm the silence has created has given rise to many menopause myths that we need to dispel.

Over the course of a year, I see hundreds of women managing the changes of peri/menopause. I'm fortunate to have conversations with them about these changes, and over the years, I've noticed most women are searching for similar understanding. As a doctor of women's health, I've learned firsthand that we can do more than just "manage." But before we can understand the inherent challenges and gifts of menopause, we must first dispel the myths that have been passed to us, either by lack of information or by misinformation, from our mothers, doctors, and friends.

To correct the myths my patients bring to my office, I often ask them to share with me what they *do* know. What have they heard from friends, doctors, mothers, sisters about the menopausal journey? They report some interesting myths.

COMMON MENOPAUSE MYTHS FROM TULA WELLNESS PATIENTS:

- "Menopause is when some or most parts of us shrivel up and die."

- "I'm not there yet, but I'm sure my vagina will turn into a tortilla."

- "Menopause is the beginning of the end."

- "You're too young to be perimenopausal in your forties. Menopause symptoms start in your fifties."

- "Decreasing estrogen is the main menopause culprit."

- "If you have had a diagnosis of cancer, you can never take hormone replacement therapy."

As you can see from my patients' responses, there are myriad myths about menopause. With so much misinformation and lack of information, there is no wonder many of us enter this stage blindly.

Above all the myths, most of us believe in the one big one: "Menopause is the beginning of the end." I hear this more often than any of the others. So many of us think of menopause as an end, as opposed to the new beginning that it is. When we approach menopause believing in this myth, we are unprepared and lacking control. We're going in not understanding what is going to happen and if or when we'll come out of it.

MYTH

Menopause is the beginning of the end.

REALITY

Menopause is the beginning of the most powerful
and transformative stage of life. Armed with
knowledge and guidance, you can harness this
innate power to live your most authentic life.

Anytime we feel like we have no control, we feel fear and unease. The reality of the menopause journey, however, is that, though bumpy, it is a wonderful time of transition and empowerment. I am the first to admit that it is hard work, not because your hormones are changing, but because you're entering the second half of your life. You're being honest with yourself, taking inventory of who you are, and manifesting your authenticity. You're letting go of who you *were* and embracing who you *are*. Menopause allows you the opportunity to unravel and recreate yourself, so that you walk into the second half of life stronger and more authentic.

Another popular myth about menopause is when it actually happens. Menopause is defined as twelve months without menstruating. Using this definition, menopause is actually just one day!

If you didn't write the first day of your last menstrual period down and keep up with that for the last year, then you're going to miss your menopause birthday. Once you reach that anniversary, then, technically, you're postmenopausal. The average age of menopause in the Western world is fifty-one.[3] Interestingly, the average age of menopause changes depending on where you live. In India, for example, the average age

---

3   "Menopause," Mayo Clinic, accessed May 1, 2019, https://www.mayoclinic.org/
diseases-conditions/menopause/symptoms-causes/syc-20353397.

of menopause is forty-six.[4] But here is the reality: you could very well be menopausal in your mid-forties, which means that you could be symptomatic by your late thirties or early forties.

MYTH

Menopause is the stage of life
after your period stops.

REALITY

Since menopause means twelve months
without menstruating, by definition menopause
is technically one day. After that day,
you are postmenopausal.

It is important to note here that we are discussing natural menopause that takes at least a year of transition between menstruation and cessation. On the other hand, surgical menopause, or removal of ovaries, causes immediate menopause. Removal of the uterus or a tubal ligation can also cause premature menopause. Once your ovaries are out—then BAM!—the menopause party instantly begins. Your estrogen levels go down, your progesterone and testosterone levels go down, and a host of other hormone fluctuations begin. This can obviously be jarring to the body and be a challenging transition for women and their partners.

---

4   Tripti Sharan, "The Menopause Mantra: Learn How to Enjoy a New Beginning," The Better India, accessed May 1, 2019, https://www.thebetterindia.com/124706/menopause-mantra-things-to-know/.

REALITY CHECK: PERIMENOPAUSE AND MENOPAUSE

We have already used the terms *perimenopause, menopause,* and *postmenopause,* so let's take a moment to identify the differences. In terms of symptoms, there are no significant differences between perimenopause and menopause. Rather, each term denotes the phase of the process a woman is in. Perimenopause represents the months to years that precede menopause. It's the name of the time period, not a defined state of one's health. Perimenopause is a period of one to eight years that precedes menopause. During this time, there is an increase in hormone fluctuations and a decrease in estrogen, progesterone, and, typically, testosterone. The symptoms of perimenopause are the same as what most women describe as "menopausal symptoms."

PERIMENOPAUSE

- Occurs between the ages of mid-thirties to fifty
- Menstrual cycles become erratic
- The number of ovarian follicles decreases
- Production of estrogen and progesterone decreases
- Hormones of reproduction become unbalanced

MENOPAUSE

- Menopause is twelve months without menstruation
- Average age for American women is fifty-one
- Removal of ovaries (surgical menopause) causes immediate menopause
- Removal of uterus or tubal ligation can cause menopausal symptoms due to the effect that surgery has on the blood supply

An important thing to understand is that menopause is not a singular event—you're not on one side of it or another. It's a progression, a continuation of your evolution, of your growth, and of your life. It's nothing to be afraid of; it's nothing to fear. It's a transformation a woman can embrace and come through better on the other side.

What most women don't realize is that menopause is already happening to them. It's not like you wake up one day and are post-menopausal. If you're more than forty-five years old, then you are almost certainly perimenopausal, even though you may not have recognized some of the subtle changes, which could include worsening PMS, insomnia, and irritability. It is also important to understand that you can be in your reproductive years and perimenopausal at the same time. For example, you can be fertile at age forty-two and able to become pregnant *and also* have significant perimenopausal symptoms. It's an interesting time, for sure. Most women are focused on their ability or inability to conceive, and rarely think about this important "in between" phase of life.

COMMON PERI/MENOPAUSE SYMPTOMS
- Depression/anxiety
- Increased blood pressure
- Increased cholesterol
- Vaginal dryness/itching
- Decreased memory
- Decreased attention span
- Pain during intercourse
- Urinary incontinence/frequency
- Dry, flaky skin
- Heart palpitations
- Osteoporosis
- Cholesterol changes
- Shortness of breath

- Thin skin
- Hair loss
- Wrinkles

It is often symptoms such as irritability and thought disturbances that frighten women the most. The erratic nature of hormones during this period can be likened to puberty. Hormones can fluctuate hour by hour, day by day. It's no wonder a woman may feel intensely irritable one moment and depressed the next. This is when knowledge can help ease the transition. This is why understanding menopause isn't just for the women it affects. It's important for partners, family, and even employers to understand the changes.

Based on my personal experiences, I now ask my patients, half-jokingly, "Have you had any homicidal thoughts lately?" There are countless women I've talked to with ferocious thoughts, dry vaginas, mild urinary incontinence issues, or fuzzy thinking who suffer through, thinking they're alone. It never occurs to them that these inconveniences can easily be fixed. Having some objectivity about what you are experiencing can drastically affect your perspective and can give you enough distance from your symptoms to see their effects on your thoughts and moods.

For this reason, the following chapters will help outline what you can expect from the peri/menopause years. Menopause is a systemic transition. It does not just affect one organ, and that is why its symptoms can be far reaching and seem unrelated. When we understand their relationship, however, we are assured that our bodies are undergoing normal changes. This can help ease your transition through your menopausal years, armed with knowledge and realities of the experience.

I hope to validate your experiences so that when you experience the symptoms listed previously, you will not assume you need antidepressants or antianxiety medications, as Tonya did in the opening story. These will not treat the source of your symptoms. Instead, you can be your own advocate, debunk the common myths, and understand that you are not in a dire state. You can then seek out a doctor who understands the realities of menopause and can help you to transition through this powerful phase of your life.

CLOSING TAKEAWAYS

1. One of the major myths of menopause is that it only relates to the menstrual cycle, or the end of it. In actuality, menopause is the beginning of our journey to become who we are meant to be.

2. Menopause allows you the opportunity to reinvent and recreate yourself, so that you walk into the second half of life stronger and more authentic.

3. Menopause is defined as twelve months without menstruating. Using this definition, menopause is actually just one day!

4. In terms of symptoms, there are no significant differences between perimenopause and menopause.

5. You can be in your reproductive years and perimenopausal at the same time.

CHAPTER 2

WHAT'S GOING ON DOWN THERE … AND EVERYWHERE ELSE?

I had a conversation with my seventy-eight-year-old mother recently after I received some new toys in the office for vaginal rejuvenation. I told her, "I'll treat you and you could be a guinea pig for one of my trainings." Her response was, "I don't need any of that stuff." I said, "Well, you have a vagina, and odds are it's dry, and odds are that doesn't really feel good." Though my mother was a reluctant participant, her initial response was similar to many women's when the topic of sexual health and satisfaction after menopause comes up. They experience changes and then become resigned to "what is."

For some women, vaginal dryness may not bother them, and that's fine, but taking ownership of your vaginas, embracing them, and knowing that you have a choice about your sexuality at all stages of life is empowering. It's true that we cannot fight nature—as we get older, libido goes down; sensation goes down; lubrication goes down. When this happens, many women think, *It's never going to be what it was*; but I'm here to tell you it actually can be what it was, and it should be what it was if that's what you want.

Women have suffered in silence for a long time because of the myth that we shouldn't discuss our sexuality, especially in our later years. The reality of menopause, however, is that you can reclaim your sexuality by knowing your options and making your own choices. Not for your partner, your friends, or your culture, but for yourself.

One of the biggest perimenopausal complaints is decreased libido. With age, many women don't have the same sensations or desires they had in their twenties.[5] A lot of women don't necessarily expect to feel like they did in their twenties, but they would like to have some semblance of that early vitality. Unfortunately, many women have resigned themselves to a numbed existence—this is not how it has to be! It is important to understand these changes and prepare for them, but don't stop there.

> **Keep seeking to understand your anatomy and its natural changes, and discover the new therapies that can help regain the vitality you once had.**

Keep seeking to understand your anatomy and its natural changes, and discover the new therapies that can help regain the vitality you once had.

Many women come to me asking if they're "normal." Do their vaginas look normal? Are their orgasms normal? Are their sensations normal? I encourage women to know what is normal for themselves,

---

5   Dana R. Ambler et. al., "Sexual Function in Elderly Women: A Review of Current Literature," *Reviews in Obstetrics and Gynecology* 5, no. 1 (2012), 16–27.

rather than compare themselves to others. Vaginas continue to be functional as women get older, but that doesn't mean they look the same as they did during a woman's early years. For many women, a good place to start is a quick internet search of the anatomy of the vagina. It's hard to discuss therapies and options when you are unclear about the terminology and aspects of sexual anatomy. Next, I encourage women to continue to know their bodies by self-exploration. An easy way to familiarize yourself with vaginal changes is to get a hand mirror and take a look. The hair can change, the skin color can alter, labia minora can lengthen and labia majora can sag. These are normal and natural changes.

Many medical practitioners have dismissed what happens between a woman's legs after age forty. Unfortunately, there are providers who believe that once a woman has had a hysterectomy or gone through menopause, there is no need to examine or even discuss the typical vaginal changes. This is yet another menopause myth to dispel, and is one of the most frustrating ones for me as a physician.

I've seen countless women who report that their providers have not bothered to look "down there" in years. It's as if to say, once a woman has finished childbearing, the vagina and vulva are irrelevant.

MYTH

After menopause or hysterectomy, there
is no need for pelvic exams.

REALITY

Unfortunately this myth is prevalent among patients *and*
doctors. Countless patients have presented for various
concerns with the misconception that once we are done
with childbearing and/or no longer have a uterus, there

is no need to bother with the lady parts. After hysterectomy, it is very possible that one may not require a
Pap smear (a procedure where a swab is used to scrape
cells of the cervix to screen for cervical cancer), but
the cervix is just one aspect of pelvic/vaginal health.

WHAT'S GOING ON DOWN THERE? ESTROGEN AND THE VAGINA

You cannot discuss the symptoms and changes of menopause without understanding the systemic effects that declining estrogen has on the body. As we will look at closely in this section, waning estrogen can have far-reaching impacts on all systems, not just on vaginal and sexual health. In the past, doctors have used terms like *atrophic vaginitis* or *vaginal atrophy* to discuss a woman's changing vaginal health. These terms, however, didn't encompass all of the symptoms of menopause, like the urinary symptoms, for instance. It's not only the vagina that is affected by declining estrogen, but everything in the pelvis, especially the urethra, vaginal wall, and exterior labia. Furthermore, there's an increase in urinary tract infections (UTI) and even urinary inconti-nence as a result of declining estrogen. In recent years, doctors have begun referring to these as Genital Symptoms of Menopause (GSM).

GSM includes thinning, drying, and inflammation of the vaginal wall due to declining estrogen. This can lead to pain with intercourse, and the lack of lubrication can also cause small tears in the vagina. That obviously doesn't feel good. (As we will discuss in chapter 4, there are ways to reintroduce estrogen, or even introduce other hormones that convert to estrogen.) For some women experiencing GSM, adding lubricating topical oils like coconut oil, which is anti-inflammatory, antifungal, antibacterial, and lubricating, can offer significant relief.

GENITAL SYMPTOMS OF MENOPAUSE (GSM)

- GSM occurs most often after menopause, but it can also develop during breastfeeding or at any other time your body's estrogen production declines

- Earliest symptoms are decreased vaginal lubrication, followed by other vaginal and urinary symptoms that may be exacerbated by superimposed infection

- Thinning, drying, and inflammation of the vaginal walls due to your body's declining estrogen levels

- Pain during intercourse, which can naturally decrease interest in sex

- Increase in urinary tract infections (UTI)

Even though there may be aesthetic changes that take place, the vagina can and should remain functional. When I'm having this libido conversation with patients and friends, however, I'm finding that some don't have a clear understanding of how their vaginas function. This must change. Women need to know what pleasures them and understand the nuances of their bodies.

Let's take a moment to address how the prevalence of pornography has influenced men's and women's expectations of sexual encounters. What we see on television and movies is unrealistic for most women, because most require clitoral stimulation in order to have an orgasm. Clitoral stimulation doesn't occur so easily during intercourse—unless you're really quite handy. Pun intended! Once I've explained to women that we generally have orgasms through clitoral stimulation, they have a sense of relief that nothing is wrong with them.

MYTH

Women should be able to climax through
intercourse without clitoral stimulation.

REALITY

Approximately 70 percent of women require direct
clitoral stimulation in order to reach climax.[6] There are
vaginal orgasms that originate from stimulation of the
anterior vaginal wall. This area has been described as the
G-spot or female prostate (yes it exists, keep reading).

The clitoris is a complex organ consisting of glans clitoris, corpus cavernous, crus clitoris, and bulb of the vestibule. There are also nerve fibers that run between the clitoris and the anterior vaginal wall. We have typically spoken about the G-spot as a separate entity apart from the clitoris, but this complex tissue is uniquely intertwined.

As women age, their ability to have orgasms with intercourse usually decreases. This is one reason it's important to know your body and the myriad ways to bring it pleasure. What has been described as a vaginal orgasm typically originates from the anterior vaginal wall G-spot area. The G-spot is this elusive area that you can't necessarily see with the naked eye, but we know that it has cells and tissues that are actually similar to the male prostate. There is still controversy regarding the existence of the G-spot. There are differences in where women can feel the G-spot, but most women can locate their G-spot by placing a finger into the vagina and pushing up toward the belly button in a "come hither" motion. Furthermore, most women can feel pleasure by massaging right at the opening of the vagina, just

---

6   Kim Wallen and Elizabeth A. Lloyd, "Female sexual arousal: Genital anatomy and orgasm in intercourse," *Hormones and Behavior* 59, no. 5 (May 2011), 780–792.

below the urethra. Some women sense more pleasure further up in the vaginal canal. This is why it's important to know *your* body and *your* pleasures. It's time to move beyond thinking of the G-spot as a discrete area for your partner to find, and instead embrace your full pleasure through self-exploration.

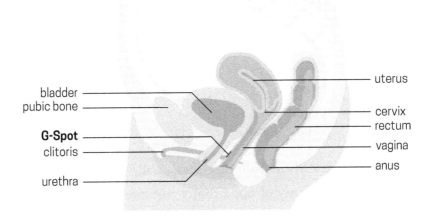

No matter the unique features of our vaginal anatomies, we need to take time exploring and figuring out how we want to experience our sexual encounters. Most women respond best to clitoral stimulation, but starting to explore the G-spot and understanding where it is and how it works can also be valuable. It's important for women to do self-exploration because we can't expect our partners to discover things we haven't discovered for ourselves. Take a mirror, take your time, and figure it out.

In addition to self-exploration, vibrators and other toys can be valuable tools for women

> It's important for women to do self-exploration because we can't expect our partners to discover things we haven't discovered for ourselves. Take a mirror, take your time, and figure it out.

learning more about their sexual pleasure. At Tula Wellness, we call them "Empowerment Tools" because we believe that knowing your body and what brings it pleasure is empowering. The dildos of today are not your mother's dildos. There are many types of vibrators on the market. Some of the best ones are clitoral and G-spot stimulators that can help a woman understand her body and can also be used during intercourse.

EMPOWERMENT TOOLS

- Clitoral vibrators
- Bullet vibrators
- Couples toys
- Realistic vibrators

I would like to remind all readers, especially those over age fifty, that there is still plenty of opportunity to explore and enjoy your sexuality. In fact, it can be a great time because you're not worrying about getting pregnant, and you may not be under the influence of certain hormones, like birth control pills, that can negatively affect your libido. At this point in life, you have the opportunity to begin exploring your sexuality in a new, liberating way. For more information on sexual health after menopause, please see the "Appendix: A Word About Vaginal Rejuvenation."

WHAT'S GOING ON WITH YOUR CHANGE IN BEHAVIOR? ESTROGEN AND THE BRAIN

At a recent health summit, an author shared with me that days prior his wife had sat down at the kitchen table with him and his daughter and presented a list of things she wasn't going to tolerate anymore. He was perplexed by her behavior. I asked how old his wife was, and he said she was in her mid-forties. I said, "Ah, she's right on schedule." Menopause can throw partners and children for a loop because they don't know what's going on. They're just trying to figure out where their wives and mothers went and if they're going to come back.

In addition to the physical changes women notice in their bodies, there are brain chemistry variations that can alter perception and personality. In a fascinating book called *The Female Brain*, neuro-psychiatrist Dr. Louann Brizendine explains how estrogen impacts a woman's outlook and emotions:

> [After menopause] the ovaries have stopped producing the hormones that have boosted her communication circuits, emotion circuits, the drive to tend and care, and the urge to avoid conflict at all costs. The circuits are still there, but the fuel for running the highly responsive Maserati engine for tracking the emotions of others has begun to run dry, and this scarcity causes a major shift in how a woman perceives her reality.... This can happen precipitously, and the problem is, [her] family can't see from the outside how her internal rules are being rewritten.[7]

As Dr. Brizendine emphasizes, estrogen is our nurturing hormone that makes us want to attend to our families. I tell my patients that estrogen is what makes you pick up dirty socks from your child's floor. As estrogen declines, however, we just aren't as interested in servitude and nurturance. One day, you find yourself saying, "Pick up your own damn socks!" Sound familiar?

As you can imagine, menopause, and the correlating brain chemistry changes, can affect family dynamics and structures. Estrogen helps you deal with some of the challenges that come with

---

7   Louann Brizendine, *The Female Brain* (New York: Morgan Road Books, 2006), 137.

being a mother and a partner. It's not just the estrogen, though; it's the Pitocin and the dopamine and all the other neurotransmitters that get activated when we're happy or see our children. But as those levels decline, there's not the same interest, or tolerance, for some aspects of mothering.

These changes can often leave our partners quite confused. When I explain to men what is happening to women, and the personality changes that might correlate, their partners nod empathically—"Yes, that sounds like my partner!" When they receive this knowledge, they gain some perspective on what women are experiencing.

If menopause is not understood, it can get pretty complicated and definitely affect relationships. Perimenopause is when the hard decisions get made. Marriages fall apart, careers change, and women begin to rediscover themselves outside of their roles within their families. I believe this has everything to do with how hormones are changing and how women are reassessing their lives and relationships. During peri/menopause, women may be a lot less tolerant and much more vocal about what they want and don't want. It's not personal against partners and families, it's a normal and natural change that needs to be discussed. These conversations are healthy ones—revolutionary ones that dispel menopause myths.

URINARY INCONTINENCE: DON'T MAKE ME LAUGH, COUGH, SNEEZE, OR JUMP!

Perhaps some of the most surprising changes that occur during peri/menopause are the ones that happen below the waist. Leakage of urine can be one of the first physiologic changes that occurs in response to hormone imbalance. In fact, 50 percent of women will have some form of stress or urge incontinence.[8] Middle age makes jumping jacks, lifting heavy objects, wheezing, and laughing quite a gamble! Even women in their thirties and early forties are experiencing incontinence, and they are altering their lives as a result of not being able to hold their urine. They often consider it a normal thing that they just accept. Some are too embarrassed to discuss it.

> 50 percent of women will have some form of stress or urge incontinence.

TYPES OF INCONTINENCE

Stress Incontinence

- Urine leaks when you exert pressure on your bladder by coughing, sneezing, laughing, exercising, or lifting something heavy

- This type is relatively easy to treat using Kegel exercises or pelvic floor strengthening devices (see the following Kegel instructions)

Urge Incontinence

- A sudden, overwhelming need to pee typically caused by spasms of the bladder muscles

- Spasms can come from nerve or muscle damage, caused by illness (like a stroke), infection, or inflammation of the bladder

- Medications and diet can worsen symptoms

- Can come on suddenly

Mixed incontinence

- A combination of stress and urge incontinences

---

8   Victor W. Nitti, "The Prevalence of Urinary Incontinence," *Reviews in Urology* 3 (2001), S2–S6.

Both stress and urge incontinence increase as we age and as estrogen levels decline. As with vaginal changes, the tissue becomes thinner and drier and doesn't function as well. At the urethra, there once was enough tissue and cells to create a plumpness so we could hold the urine easier; but as that plumpness decreases, the risk of urinary tract infections (UTI) increases because the bacteria that are present actually can ascend into the bladder more easily. This can also affect the vaginal pH. We need to keep a certain pH in order to keep a balance of flora, since the vagina has its own special group of bacteria. The pH allows certain bacteria to grow and discourages other strains of bacteria. Our vaginas usually function best when the pH is on the higher end, but as we age, pH levels decrease, making the vaginal environment more acidic.

Urge incontinence is not as easy to treat as stress, because the urge incontinence is usually due to bladder spasms. It can come on quite suddenly and is associated with poor diet, high caffeine intake, smoking, and stress. There are certainly a lot of medications that can worsen it and then other medications that improve it.

DIAGNOSING INCONTINENCE
- Medical history
- Urine sample
- Physical exam
- Diary

All forms of incontinence can be helped by good bladder hygiene and being on a schedule to empty your bladder. This sounds elementary, but as women, we're really good at holding our bladders for an incredible length of time. As we age, however, that ability goes down precipitously. So, getting into the habit of voiding on a regular basis is helpful.

MYTH

Urinary leakage is inevitable and untreatable.

REALITY

Though some changes are inevitable, there are
a variety of exercises and tools available that
diminish the severity of urinary incontinence.

Incontinence can change the quality of a woman's life. I have met women who quit exercising and doing heavy lifting to avoid incontinence. Often, however, their issues might be less about estrogen levels and more about weakening pelvic floor muscles. For this reason, strengthening the pelvic floor becomes imperative as we age.

The Pelvic Floor

The pelvic floor is a hammock-shaped muscle that attaches anteriorly/posteriorly and on each side of the pelvis. It assists in our ability to hold urine and stool, supports the back and the abdominal organs, and even impacts the intensity of our orgasms. As you can see, it's a win-win strategy to strengthen these muscles.

One of the easiest (and cheapest!) ways to strengthen your pelvic floor is through Kegel exercises. There are different things you can do to remind yourself to perform these exercises. Some women do it when they're at stoplights. Some women do it while they're in the shower. Find the time of day that works for you. The best part it, nobody even knows you're doing it!

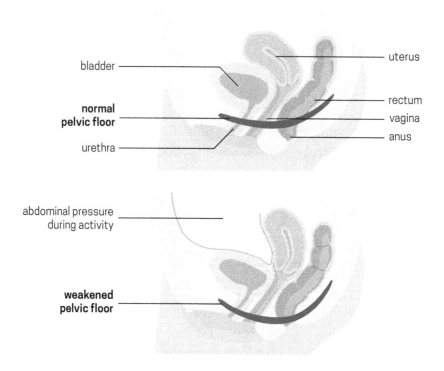

KEGEL MUSCLE STRENGTHENING EXERCISE

- To engage your Kegel muscle, you want to contract it anteriorly. Imagine that you have to urinate and you're trying to stop it; squeeze that muscle as hard as you can. Feel that? That is the anterior pelvic floor.

- The posterior pelvic floor, where the rectum is, is connected but is a slightly different muscle. The way to contract that muscle is to imagine that you have the sensation of a bowel movement that you don't want to have, so you squeeze your rectal muscles to stop a bowel movement. That is the posterior pelvic floor.

- Do these exercises once a day and you will begin to strengthen your pelvic floor, thus decreasing urinary incontinence and increasing sexual pleasure.

In addition to Kegel exercises, there are many products and therapies available to strengthen the pelvic floor. Some include beads and weighted balls. There are also vibrators that vibrate to cue you to contract your pelvic floor. See, doing Kegels can also be fun! For a note on vaginal rejuvenation's role in aiding incontinence, please see the appendix at the end of the book. If you are really suffering from urinary incontinence, you should consider seeing a specialist in pelvic floor rehabilitation. Pelvic floor rehabilitation is essentially physical therapy for your pelvic floor. Many patients remain dumbfounded by Kegel exercises. For some pelvic floor conditions, Kegels are actually contraindicated.

WHAT'S GOING ON EVERYWHERE ELSE?

Other peri/menopause complaints can be even more serious and affect our health in a myriad of ways, including memory, depression, insomnia, and osteoporosis. I don't want you to be surprised by the effects of aging, so, let's take a look at these complaints—both big and small—that are a natural part of the aging process.

Female Pattern Hair Loss

Hair loss (alopecia) can be one of the most distressing signs of aging. Up to two-thirds of postmenopausal women will be affected with some form. Stress, medications, and medical conditions can contribute. Hypothyroidism, hormone imbalances, PCOS (polycystic ovarian syndrome), and nutritional deficiencies are all culprits.

In my personal experience, perimenopause can mean losing hair in places you want it, and growing hair in places you don't, like my chin hair and its increasing number of cohorts! One of the most common complaints I hear from women is about thinning hair, especially in the front and the crown of their heads. First and foremost, I would say it is important in this situation to look at hormones. Although they may not be predictive, they will at least help you look into other reasons why you could be losing hair—one of the most common causes being thyroid dysfunction (which we will discuss fully in chapter 5). The increase in unwanted hair and the decrease in desired hair is also associated with hormone fluctuations, declining estrogen, and the ratio between estrogen and testosterone. Though some cases can be caused by genetics, some can be mitigated by balancing hormones.

The initial work-up includes an analysis of hormones, complete blood count, and iron levels.

Medications such as Minoxidil can be helpful but unfortunately require continued application or hair loss will reoccur. Anti androgen medications such as spironolactone can also be helpful but come with their own host of side effects. I have seen some success in my practice with the injection of platelet-rich plasma (growth factors) under the scalp, inducing collagen, to stimulate hair growth.

This is one of the more popular treatments in the office. Finally, hair transplantation is definitely an option that works well. Many women have found great success with them.

We all have the "chin hair in the mirror" story. As we get older, we add new stories and grievances—like dry skin, thinning hair, and a spare tire. So let's keep the party going and look at more of the changes women experience after age thirty-five.

Osteoporosis

During the first five to ten years of menopause, women lose the most amount of bone. The recommendation (at the time of printing) by The American College of Obstetricians and Gynecologists is that woman entering menopause consider hormone therapy for the first five years, unless contraindicated.

MYTH

Estrogen is only for controlling hot flashes.

REALITY

Taking estrogen in the first three to five years of menopause can reduce bone loss by 30 percent.[9]

In addition to hormone therapy, or in place of it if you can't take hormone therapy, maintain an appropriate diet and supplement with vitamin D and calcium. It's important to note that calcium can't do its job if your vitamin D is inadequate, so ask your doctor for a simple blood test to ensure that your vitamin D levels are no less than thirty. I ideally like vitamin D3 levels to be between fifty and seventy-five. As for calcium, too much is not a good thing. You should attempt to get calcium through the foods listed below as much as you can.

CALCIUM-RICH FOODS
- Kefir
- Broccoli
- Almonds
- Okra
- Navy Beans
- Cheese
- Yogurt

Another powerful way to protect your bones is through weight-bearing exercises. This doesn't mean you have to become a bodybuilder

9 ACOG Practice Bulletin Number 129, September 2012 (Replaces Practice Bulletin No. 50, January 2004) (Reaffirmed 2019).

(though if you do, your bones might thank you). Even low-impact exercises like walking, tai chi, and yoga count as great bone-strengthening exercises.

Heart Palpitations

Another symptom I want to briefly mention is heart palpitations. Palpitations are a common symptom that sends women into emergency rooms each day. As estrogen levels fall and fluctuate, it's extremely common to experience heart palpitations. This symptom is generally relieved with estrogen treatment, but it can be quite unsettling if you do not know to expect it.

Brain Fog

Brain fog, or cotton brain, as some of us lovingly refer to it, can be alarming. As I mentioned earlier, one of my most profound menopausal experiences was during a surgery I had performed more than a thousand times. I remember looking at the inside of my patient's abdomen and thinking, *What next?* Don't make light of this symptom. It can be life changing. I remember seeing people I had known for years, and not remembering their names. It was scary and embarrassing until I realized what was happening. You can go from being a very high-functioning person to feeling like you are in the early stages of dementia or Alzheimer's disease. The inability to recall words, the names of long-term friends, and why you wandered into the next room is unnerving and frightening. There are multiple factors including adrenal fatigue, leaky gut, and blood sugar imbalances that contribute to mental clarity.

Insomnia

Insomnia is another common complaint of perimenopause and beyond. The importance of sleep cannot be overstated. There is a strong link to sleep disturbances and multiple health issues, including:

- Weight gain
- Elevated cholesterol
- Diabetes
- Hormone imbalance

Often, women will have the ability to fall asleep, but then they wake up at 3:00 a.m. and can't go back to sleep. Unfortunately, insomnia tends to get worse with aging, and there are many factors that affect your ability to fall asleep. Obviously, our exposure to electronic devices and what we have on our minds before we get into bed can set the tone for our sleep quality. Decreasing estrogen levels can contribute to night sweats that can be mild to severe, causing women to wake up in a pool of sweat. Changing clothes and sheets in the middle of the night can certainly make it tough to get the rest we need.

Another culprit of insomnia is alcohol, especially wine. Sorry, ladies! Increased alcohol intake can definitely affect your ability to sleep. For many women, simply adjusting their alcohol intake can solve their sleep disturbances.

Obstructive Sleep Apnea (OSA) can worsen during menopause, as estrogen and progesterone levels decline. OSA is a condition where breathing temporarily pauses during sleep. The decreased oxygen affects brain, hormones, and cardiac health. Many patients go undiagnosed from this very serious condition. Consider asking your provider to order a sleep study if you suspect you are affected.

SIGNS THAT YOU MAY HAVE OSA

- Loud snoring
- Daytime sleepiness
- Difficulty concentrating
- Morning headache
- Abrupt waking during sleep and/or observed episodes of breathing cessation

There are, of course, many sleep aids, supplements, and medications for insomnia. Hormone therapy can drastically improve your sleep as well.

Progesterone is a hormone that's calming and can also alleviate some of the anxiety symptoms of perimenopause.

NATURAL PROGESTERONE FOR SLEEP

For women having difficulty with sleep, natural progesterone can be a useful medication. But when you say "I can't sleep," I need to know more than that. Do you have problems falling asleep or staying asleep? Are you waking up with your mind racing or are you waking up alert? Depending on your answer to that, it could be a lack of estrogen, a lack of progesterone, or actually too much cortisol. Patients with high cortisol levels are what I call "wired and tired." People with estrogen imbalance deficiency usually can't sleep because they wake up with hot flashes. People with the progesterone deficiency usually have a hard time going to sleep and staying asleep. So, depending on the specifics of your sleep disturbances, hormonal therapy (see chapter 4) might be right for you. Check with your doctor for more information.

Depression and Anxiety

If you have a history of depression and/or anxiety, it's very possible you will experience it again as you go through perimenopause. For this reason, the forties can be quite challenging for many women. Often, you'll find that your normal coping mechanisms just aren't helping anymore. No, you aren't crazy. You're normal. Anxiety is one of the more common complaints I hear. There are many factors potentially affecting anxiety, including decreasing progesterone and overactive adrenal activity. I wish I had the magic bullet to offer here but there is none. Many of the treatments discussed throughout the book address this common symptom. I encourage patients to take a serious look at their gut health and diet as a means to combat their depression and anxiety. We will discuss therapies throughout the book and deal with gut health in chapter 6.

***

As we can see by the varied topics of this chapter, declining estrogen can have systemic effects on our bodies. From hair loss to mood swings, from bladder leakage to weakened bones, waning estrogen levels have powerful effects on women's bodies. Understand that when you experience the seemingly disparate symptoms discussed in this chapter, you are undergoing the normal changes that come with aging. They do not have to rule your life or alter it drastically, but they do encourage you to take an active, engaged role in your own evolution. This is not an exhaustive review of all symptoms. Receding gum lines, persistent, chronic itch (pruritus), and ringing in the ears (tinnitus) are all also on the long list of unsuspecting symptoms you may experience. As we will discuss in later chapters, diet and lifestyle changes can mitigate many of the inconvenient symptoms discussed in this chapter.

CLOSING TAKEAWAYS

1. Decreased libido is a common complaint of perimenopause.

2. Waning estrogen can have far-reaching impacts on all systems, not just on vaginal and sexual health. Nevertheless, there is still plenty of opportunity to explore and enjoy your sexuality.

3. In addition to the physical changes women notice in their bodies, there are brain chemistry variations that can alter perception and personality.

4. Leakage of urine can be one of the first physiologic changes that occurs in response to hormone imbalance. Both stress and urge incontinences increase as we age and as estrogen levels decline.

5. Other peri/menopause complaints can be even more serious and affect our health in myriad ways, including memory, depression, insomnia, and osteoporosis.

CHAPTER 3

SEX HORMONES 101

Here's what you need to know in a nutshell: hormones can be a bitch. That's pretty much the bottom line. I'm not here to sugarcoat hormonal changes or the effects they can have on a woman's life, but I am here to inform and validate. This chapter will serve as an informational and foundational piece on which later treatment chapters will build. We will dispel many of the common myths that women and doctors often hold about the complex issue of hormones.

Surprisingly, women don't know much about their hormones, and yet hormones affect the prism through which we see the world and ourselves. Notwithstanding the underdeveloped prefrontal cortex, hormones play a role in your teenager's behavior and why you may only want to have sex with your partner one day out of the month (ovulation). Hormones can intensify our rage, sadness, empathy—you name it. If we've gone through half our lives not understanding our hormones, then how are we to make sense of them in the second half of life? Let's get the conversation started.

We've been going through the change since birth, and we're therefore constantly adapting to hormonal fluctuations. So, interestingly, when we are menopausal our hormones are more like they were in our prepubescent state. All of our hormone levels are much lower, and eventually they get back down to that prepubescent baseline. From puberty through reproduction, and then through perimenopause, we are constantly going through some fluctuation or transition into the next phase. Puberty is the transition from the prepubescent to reproductive phase. We spend a lot of time in the reproductive stage, but with life expectancies into our eighties, we actually spend more time in the premenopausal and menopausal phases. Those phases are similar to puberty in terms of the hormonal fluctuations; but this time around, we might have jobs, partners, children, or other responsibilities to manage while dealing with hormonal fluctuations. For this reason, things can get quite messy in our later years.

The following graphic shows how our estrogen levels diminish slightly over time, rather than our experiencing an immediate decrease in estrogen. Levels rise back up to a normal baseline, but it's really the acute drops in estrogen that cause symptoms such as hot flashes.

LIFE CYCLE OF OVARIAN HORMONES

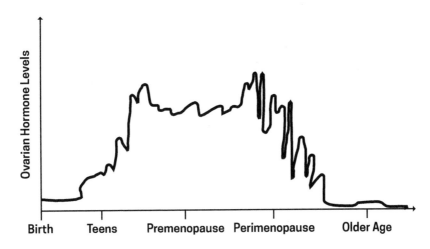

One common misconception is that you need to get your hormones checked to confirm that you're perimenopausal. I do think you should have them checked, but you're not checking them to define whether there is an issue. You're checking them to get a baseline. News flash: your hormones can look completely normal and you can still be in the throes of perimenopause. Normal hormone levels mean nothing to the perimenopausal woman. Disappearing hormones don't dictate whether you're going to have symptoms of weight gain and hair loss, irritability, mood swings, and worsening PMS; they're all going to still happen and your hormones can look entirely normal.

MYTH

Getting your hormones checked will
determine if you are perimenopausal.

REALITY

Symptoms are the best determinant of
your peri/menopause symptoms.

A lot of patients say, "I want to get my hormones checked because I think something is going on." Then I say, "We can check your hormones, but your hormones aren't the indicator of something going on. If you're forty-five, something is going on! I don't need to check your hormones to tell you that, because your hormones are fluctuating all the time." I do draw the hormones, but it is so we have a baseline. In the event that anything is abnormal, we can address it. But mostly, if we decide at some later point to start hormones, we know where you are naturally. I usually try to just treat symptoms, not lab results. Once your symptoms are better, that indicates that your hormones are better.

Again, your hormones can look totally fine even though you're a hot mess, or they can look really bad, but you feel fine and you're not having any hot flashes. So, you don't "need" hormone levels checked to validate your perimenopausal status. It's really more about how you're feeling. Trust your body and its symptoms, and make sure to find a doctor who will do the same.

There is one hormone, follicle stimulating hormone (FSH), that can indicate whether a woman is menopausal. FSH is produced in an area in the brain called the *anterior pituitary*. It senses how much estrogen we have. As our estrogen levels go down, the brain is stimulated to produce more FSH. FSH then alerts the ovaries to produce more estrogen. That's why we can sometimes use FSH levels to confirm menopausal state. If a woman's FSH is over thirty and she has not had a menstrual cycle for one year, then she is in menopause. However, a woman can have what seems to be a relatively normal FSH until she is definitely postmenopausal, so it's not a clear indication of whether a woman is in perimenopause.

SEX HORMONES AND THE MENSTRUAL CYCLE

There are three sex hormones that are working in concert with each other. Estrogen, which is produced primarily in the ovaries, has three types: estrone (E1), estradiol (E2), and estriol (E3). Each hormone is important, though this varies depending on which stage of life we're in. *Estrone*, for example, is the strongest estrogen, and it is primarily produced around menopause. This hormone is thought to have more of the negative effects on our health. *Estradiol* is the most prevalent form of estrogen in the body and is primarily produced in the premenopausal woman. When we take a hormone replacement, including birth control, estradiol is typically the estrogen that we use. *Estriol* is usually found in the body during pregnancy and is derived from the placenta to support fetal growth and development. All three of these types of estrogen work together with progesterone and testosterone. There are many other hormones, but for the purpose of our discussion, we will focus on these three.

SEX HORMONES

- **Estrogen**
  - Estrone (E1)—converted from estradiol
  - Estradiol (E2)—ovary—premenopausal
  - Estriol (E3)—placenta—pregnancy

- **Progesterone**

- **Testosterone**

The menstrual cycle is a microcosm of a woman's whole environment, and that environment is built by the above hormones working in concert. In the normal menstruating woman, follicles within the ovaries produce a certain amount of estrogen. Once a woman ovulates, the corpus luteum, which is a cyst that forms in the ovary at mid-cycle, produces progesterone. Progesterone is the balancer of estrogen and is required for pregnancy continuation.

Estrogen is the hormone that builds up the lining of the uterine wall, and progesterone is the hormone that opposes estrogen and allows for that lining to be broken down, thus producing menstruation. But as we go into perimenopause, we're no longer ovulating at the same rate. So we are continuing to make estrogen, but we are not having that same counterbalance with the progesterone.

MYTH

Low estrogen is the main cause of
perimenopausal symptoms.

REALITY

Low progesterone is the main culprit as women enter perimenopause. Our cycles become more erratic, in part because we are no longer ovulating consistently and, therefore, are not producing progesterone. Low progesterone is the culprit linked to worsening PMS, anxiety, insomnia, irritability, and irregular menstrual cycles.

When there are imbalances in the aforementioned hormones, things can get complicated. This is when it becomes so important for a woman to maintain body awareness so she can assist her doctor in navigating her particular imbalances. These imbalances arise from having too little of a particular hormone—a deficiency—or too much of a hormone—a dominance. A woman can present with symptoms of estrogen dominance, estrogen deficiency, progesterone dominance, progesterone deficiency, or testosterone deficiency.

SYMPTOMS OF HORMONE IMBALANCE[10]

Symptoms of Estrogen Deficiency

- Thinning skin
- Vaginal dryness
- Dry skin
- Heart palpitations
- Hot flashes
- Inability to reach climax

Symptoms of Testosterone Deficiency

- Thinning skin
- Vaginal dryness
- Blunted motivation
- Fatigue
- Diminished feeling of well-being

Symptoms of Progesterone Deficiency

- Anxiety
- Cramping
- Insomnia
- Irregular menses
- Joint pain
- Irritability
- Mood swings

PMS

- Swollen breasts
- Weight gain

---

10 Adapted from: John R. Lee, Jesse Hanley, and Virginia Hopkins, *What Your Doctor May Not Tell You About Premenopause: Balancing Your Hormones and Your Life from Thirty to Fifty* (New York: Warner Books, 1999).

Symptoms of Estrogen, Progesterone, or Testosterone Deficiencies

- Depression
- Fuzzy thinking
- Hair loss
- Headaches
- Irritability
- Low sex drive
- Memory lapses
- Inability to focus

Symptoms of Estrogen Dominance

- Fatigue
- Breast tenderness
- Fluid retention
- Craving sweets
- Decreased libido
- Heavy/irregular periods
- Mood swings
- Fibrocystic breasts
- Uterine fibroids
- Loss of scalp hair
- Sleep disturbances
- Weight gain
- Headache

There is definitely overlap in estrogen deficiency and estrogen dominance—likewise with progesterone deficiency and progesterone dominance. There are some hallmark signs, however, which is why it's so important to notice your symptoms and for doctors to take those symptoms seriously. Perimenopausal symptoms are often caused by progesterone deficiency. When you get closer to menopause or are postmenopausal, however, estrogen deficiency becomes more of an issue. When you're perimenopausal, you're not ovulating as frequently. That's why your cycles become more irregular. A hallmark sign of estrogen deficiency—and it's really not even that your estrogen is deficient; it's just there are moments when your estrogen has a steep decline—is when your symptoms include hot flashes. You can expect your estrogen levels to slowly decline as you hit your official post-menopausal years.

Perhaps the most misunderstood hormone is testosterone. Testosterone, often considered a male hormone, is actually just as important in women. In fact, women make approximately ten times more testosterone than estrogen. Most people think of testosterone as the hormone responsible for libido, but it does a lot more than just increase libido. Testosterone is important for our bones, muscle strength, and energy. It also helps with overall motivation and drive.

MYTH

Testosterone is a male hormone. Women make more estrogen daily than testosterone.

REALITY

Doctors and patients alike are misguided about the role and importance of testosterone. Women make up to ten times more testosterone than estrogen. Whereas the vagina canal is more sensitive to estrogen, the outer vaginal tissue (vulva and introitus) is more sensitive to testosterone.

TREATING THE SYMPTOMS

Once I gather information about a woman's symptoms and identify what hormones are dominant or deficient, I don't just offer hormones to fix the problem. There are definitely other treatments available. In fact, one of the most powerful things you can do to mitigate the symptoms of perimenopause is to alter your diet and lifestyle. Stress, sugar, and inflammatory foods exacerbate all of the issues that you may already be having. So if you are already having hot flashes and then you start drinking red wine, eating certain foods, or being in warm environments, then you're going to aggravate the problem. Because this is such an important component to overall health, we will explore them fully in later chapters to learn about the practical, daily things you can do to ease your symptoms.

***

As you can see, hormones can get daunting, not only for the patient, but even for the doctor. All doctors have a general understanding of how hormones work. The devil is in the details of hormonal fluctuations, and most medical training does not delve into the subtleties. Most conventional doctors aren't trained in the nuances of hormone balances. This has allowed for many menopausal myths to circulate, which in turn negatively impacts women's peri/menopausal years. This is why it is so important to pay attention to your body and what is "normal" for you—that is the greatest reality you have. Just as it's important to know yourself sexually, so it's important to notice your physical and emotional symptoms. Despite how complicated hormones can be, let this chapter be a reminder that you don't need a medical degree to observe your symptoms and let them guide you through these hormonal imbalances. Continue discussing the realities of your menopausal experience with your doctor, your friends, and your daughters.

CLOSING TAKEAWAYS

1. Disappearing hormones don't dictate whether you're going to have symptoms of weight gain and hair loss, irritability, mood swings, and worsening PMS; they're all going to still happen and your hormones can look entirely normal.

2. Maintain body awareness so you can assist your practitioner in navigating your particular hormone imbalances.

3. Diet and lifestyle changes can have the greatest impact on perimenopausal symptoms. Stress, sugar, and inflammatory foods exacerbate peri/menopausal symptoms.

CHAPTER 4

GETTING RELIEF

Samantha presented at my clinic as a hot mess. She came to the office with her husband, who sat silently as his wife described all of her symptoms—she felt she had been "deteriorating" for the past several years, and more recently felt that she was "losing her mind." She had anxiety, depression, and was barely functioning at her job as an accountant. Her marriage was also starting to . . . *Ah, I've heard that before*, I thought during our meeting. . . . rted crying gently, before it turned into full blown bawl. . . . pt to pull herself together, she couldn't, so her . . . ly while she cried. "I need help," she begged.

. . . patient, I would take an integrative . . . the Food Elimination Diet and . . . management techniques; but . . . cy. There was nothing to be . . . iate help. On that first visit, I . . . none levels and then advised her . . . e supplements immediately. I knew that she did not have the presence of mind or fortitude to follow the usual integrative medical approach. I said, "You're going to come back in three weeks and then we're going to have a conversation."

When she returned, she was feeling better, and we were able to have conversations about her diet and lifestyle. One of the reason's Samantha's case was so memorable to me was because, firstly, she was one of two patients that I have prescribed hormones on their first visit because of their dire circumstances, and secondly, because several months later her husband hand-delivered a letter to me. He cried as he handed it to me and thanked me for giving him back his wife. Everybody in my office was in tears. It was a wonderful reminder that we really are helping people.

Two months into treatment, Samantha returned as a completely different woman. She was almost unrecognizable. Since that time, she has brought in her mother and her friend, both in similar situations. She did eventually do the Food Elimination Diet and lost twenty pounds. Her husband did the diet with her and also lost weight. They changed their whole lifestyle, and the entire family benefited from this one woman asking for help and empowering herself to accept what was offered. We couldn't start with extreme lifestyle change, but in the end we were able to get back to that.

I use this case as an atypical example of how I approach patients. As much as I know that Hormone Replacement Therapy (HRT) ca be life-changing for some women, I am not a hormone push always want to start by getting an idea of the patient's lifesty diet, and then honing in on their hormonal needs, if any; b now and then, there's a patient who is just so miserable that immediate relief of her symptoms.

Like Samantha, some women have extreme responses for others, this time is merely a challenging inconveni where you fall on that spectrum, it's important to pay attention to your body and ask for help when you are struggling. The doctor's office should be a safe space where you can ask for support if you need it. If you don't feel comfortable asking for your doctor's aid, it might be an indication that you need a different practitioner.

MEASURING HORMONES

I'm often asked *how* you should get your hormones checked: through urine, saliva, or blood? All of these methods have potential benefits, but if you are on hormone replacement, one of the best ways to evaluate your levels is through a twenty-four-hour urine collection, because it collects the total amount of hormones over a full day as opposed to getting a spot evaluation of your hormones through blood testing. The salivary hormones, on the other hand, can be convenient for checking your natural hormone levels, and there is evidence that they can be more specific, but not once you're on hormone therapy. Traditional gynecologists will typically draw your blood and there are some providers who don't even measure hormones. Don't get caught up in trying to measure the moving target, your hormones. Your symptoms are always first and foremost the indicator of what's happening. (See the Resources section for available options.)

HORMONE REPLACEMENT THERAPY

Nobody makes HRT easy for the patients (or most doctors) to understand. I don't believe that every woman should be on HRT, and I certainly don't believe that women should be menstruating into their seventies and eighties. However, I do believe that when supplementation is appropriate, the body should recognize the hormone—as in a bioidentical hormone. When you hear the term *bioidentical hormones*, it simply means they are the same molecular composition as what your body naturally makes.

MYTH

Bioidentical hormones are safer
than synthetic hormones.

REALITY

Bioidentical hormones carry the same risk
as synthetic hormones. Bioidentical hormones
have the identical molecular structure of
hormones that your body makes.

It's often a challenge to talk about bioidentical hormones because there is so much controversy, and the FDA has been slow to approve them. I remember a conversation I had with a doctor several years ago on the topic of my bioidentical hormones. She said she thought that bioidentical hormones were a "publicity stunt." I must confess that I used to be one of those conventional doctors who doubted these new advancements in HRT, but I now recognize that although conventional medicine has certainly created amazing opportunities for health and healing, it is still behind in the area of hormone replacement, especially as it pertains to women.

MYTH

Compounding pharmacies are the only
way to get bioidentical hormones.

REALITY

There are many FDA-approved bioidentical medications
on the market, including estrogen and progesterone.
Your doctor can write you a prescription for bioidentical
hormones that you can get from your local pharmacy.

This is what makes a conversation about bioidentical hormones challenging and full of myths. Conventional medicine might argue that there is no scientific evidence that consuming a bioidentical drug is not superior to other formulations derived from pregnant horses. I'm not here to argue any point, so decide for yourself what makes more sense for you. Despite whether you chose bioidentical hormones or synthetic, the three most common hormones that we try to balance through hormone replacement and supplementation are estrogen, progesterone, and testosterone. If you're going to replace a hormone, it makes sense to replace it as closely to the one that your body already produces.

A Note on Compounding Pharmacies

You will also hear about compounding pharmacies when you discuss HRT with your doctor. One of the trickiest aspects of prescribing hormones to patients is the role of compounding pharmacies. These pharmacies have been used for decades, but in recent years there has been some scrutiny about their practices. In 2012, a compounding pharmacy made headlines because they sent out products that weren't sterile, thus resulting in 750 cases of fungal meningitis, including sixty-four deaths. Since that time, there has been a focus on making sure that these pharmacies are delivering products that are safe. Most recently, the FDA has advanced the oversight of compounding pharmacies and created new regulatory measures through the Drug Quality and Security Act (DQSA). All of the products used at the compounding pharmacy are FDA-approved products, but the combination of them is what is not FDA approved. Compounding pharmacies use FDA-approved components, but by the time they combine them in any concentration, it becomes a new drug that has not been subject to the FDA scrutiny. Although compounding pharmacies play an integral role in the creation and distribution of bioidentical hormones, it is important to do your research before enlisting one, in order to keep you and your family safe.

Safety of Hormone Replacement Therapy

The landmark 2002 Women's Health Initiative (WHI) study perhaps offered as much confusion to our understanding hormones as it offered clarity. The study was designed to look at the risk/benefit of estrogen and progesterone for chronic disease prevention in postmenopausal women. The study results prompted many medical professionals to buy into a myth, and consequently withhold hormone replacement therapy from countless women. Prior to the study, at least 40 percent of postmenopausal women in the United States were taking HRT.[11] After the study, estrogen became the enemy, and millions of women were taken off of their supplementation. Patients were told that it was the culprit causing cardiovascular disease, breast cancer, stroke, and blood clots.

The study was ultimately flawed, however, and has since been redacted and reanalyzed because the original study looked at the

---

11   Roger A. Lobo, "Where Are We 10 Years After the Women's Health Initiative?" *J Clin Endocrinol & Metab.* 98, no. 5 (May 2013): 1771–1780. doi: 10.1210/ jc.2012-4070. Epub Mar 14, 2013.

effects of starting hormones in women who had no previous exposure to hormones; for example, they were starting women in their sixties on estrogen. That is not the way we would do hormone replacement now. If you're going to have hormone replacement, it's probably going to benefit you most in your mid-forties to your mid-fifties. We know that during that period, hormones are generally considered safe, especially if you're taking a low dose for a short period of time.

MYTH

Taking estrogen during perimenopause/early menopause will increase my risk of breast cancer.

REALITY

The safest time to take estrogen and/or progesterone is in the perimenopausal period for the shortest duration as possible (five to eight years). Women who initiate HRT within ten years of menopause and under age sixty are at the lowest risk.[12]

As you can see, there is much debate in the medical community about who should be on HRT and who should not. We also know that hormones are protective of bone health in the first few years of menopause. Even if you don't have any symptoms of menopause, you might benefit if you have a risk factors or history of osteoporosis in the family.

It is important to see a provider who has your long-term health in mind. Most women can manage menopausal symptoms through diet, lifestyle, and supplements. However, HRT can be a lifesaver for

---

12   North American Menopause Society, "The 2017 Hormone Therapy Position Statement of The North American Menopause Society," *Menopause* 24, no. 7 (July 2017): 728–53. doi: 10.1097/GME.0000000000000921.

women such as Samantha with debilitating peri/menopausal symptoms. The goal of hormone replacement is to give you the lowest dose for the least amount of time. For some women, that can be a year or two. For others, we try to start decreasing their dose as soon as possible. When deciding if HRT is right for you, consider your "quality of life" and weigh this against the potential risk.

> # When deciding if HRT is right for you, consider your "quality of life" and weigh this against the potential risk.

There are only a handful of medical schools and ob-gyn residencies that fully address the multiple issues arising for women who have passed their reproductive years. In the meantime, there are many providers functioning under longstanding myths about HRT and how to manage this large section of the population.

MYTH

With a history of breast cancer, I have no options for the relief of vaginal symptoms.

REALITY

There are multiple products on the market for the relief of vaginal dryness. On average, estrogen cream can be used in the vagina without significant systemic absorption. For people who are advised against estrogen or don't want to take estrogen, DHEA may be an option. DHEA breaks down to estrogen and testosterone on a local cellular level in the vaginal tissue.

If you are considering HRT, you should weigh the consequences and compare quality of life versus potential side effects. In other words, don't avoid hormones because you think they *might* cause cancer. Don't fall prey to the menopause myths. Do your research and discover the realities. If you're miserable, then what kind of life are you living? Even if a drug therapy has a theoretical risk, it's not a risk for every person the same way. Genetics, diet, and toxic exposures all play integral roles. Estrogen in and of itself isn't always the culprit.

In the end, the decision whether or not to use HRT is personal and directly related to a patient's quality of life. For some, HRT can be the difference between living your best life or suffering through it. It's not an easy road to navigate, which is why it is so important to be an informed patient who understands your family history, exposures, and risk factors.

A Word About HRT for Vaginal Dryness

One of the main symptoms of menopause that women experience is vaginal dryness. You don't need to take a systemic hormone for vaginal dryness. You can just take a suppository or a cream and apply it locally. You will not get the same systemic impact you would get if you were taking a pill or a patch. Furthermore, some women suffering from dryness get relief from dehydroepiandrosterone (DHEA), which is a hormone produced in the adrenal glands that breaks down into estrogen and testosterone in the body. It has been compounded for years as a suppository to treat vaginal dryness, and it works well. Within the last couple of years, the FDA-approved Prasterone (Intrarosa) for vaginal dryness and pain with intercourse, and it is generally considered safe for women who have a history of breast cancer. If you have a complicated health history or previous disease, such as breast cancer, then you are going to have to find a practitioner who will be willing to work with you. You need close monitoring if you choose hormonal treatments. As always, be an informed patient and talk with your physician before beginning any new treatments.

TREATMENT OPTIONS

In addition to HRT, there are a number of other treatments that can have positive effects on the symptoms of menopause. As always, consult with your doctor and do your research to find the therapy, or combination thereof, that best treats your symptoms.

Hormone-Balancing Supplements and Botanicals

There are quite a few supplements and botanicals that can be helpful during menopause, listed below. There are two, however, that I find to be particularly important. One that I prescribe often is Chaste Berry (Vitex), which is useful in the metabolism and production of progesterone. Women who are experiencing worsening PMS can benefit from this supplement, as well as those who are anovulatory (meaning you just don't ovulate with every menstrual cycle or you may not ovulate at all), because it helps to regulate the menstrual cycle. It is also helpful with the early symptoms associated with perimenopause. I usually start younger women (thirty-five to forty) on Chaste Berry to help with progesterone balance.

The other supplement I want to highlight is vitamin D, which is important for hormones to work. A lot of women present with vitamin D deficiencies. When we correct those levels through supplementation, sometimes their symptoms cease. For this reason, it's important to have your vitamin D levels checked, and increase them if needed.

Hormone Balancing Supplements and Botanicals:

- Chaste Berry (Vitex agnus castus)

- Black Cohosh (Actaea racemosa, Cimicifuga racemosa)

- Siberian rhubarb

- St. John's wort (Hypericum perforatum)

- Kava (Piper methysticum)

- Hops (humulus lupulus)

- Sage (Salvia officinalis)

Birth Control Pills for Menopause

Birth control pills do not contain natural progesterone. They contain progestin (synthetic progesterone), which in some cases have the opposite effect of its natural counterpart. For this reason, I don't prescribe birth control for menopausal women. Most fifty-year-old women aren't going to get pregnant. If you're concerned about pregnancy in the later years, then you can confirm your infertility by evaluating your follicle stimulating hormone levels (FSH). Specifically, if your FSH is above fifty, then there is essentially no opportunity for spontaneous pregnancy. During this stage of life, when women are no longer ovulating and creating the progesterone to counterbalance the effects of the estrogen, irregular bleeding is common.

MYTH

Oral contraceptive pills (OCPs) have no effect
on your hormonal or sexual health.

REALITY

OCPs contain synthetic estrogens and progestins and
are one of the most influential drugs women are exposed
to during their reproductive years. Approximately
70 percent of women take oral contraception in their
lifetimes.[13] OCPs can have a significant impact on
women's psychiatric health, with up to 30 percent higher
incidence of depression and a significant impact on sex
hormones, especially estrogen and testosterone.[14]

IUD for Menopause

Some providers will prescribe progestin containing IUDs for perimenopausal patients, to counteract women's naturally waning progesterone production. This progestin acts locally on the uterine lining,
and does what IUDs in general do, which is create a hostile environment for an embryo so it can't implant. I have had patients, however,
who feel the systemic impact of that progestin-containing IUD. For
some women, it might work well and help with irregular bleeding,
but for others it comes with a host of unwelcome side effects.

---

13 Kimberly Daniels, Ph.D., and Joyce C. Abma, Ph.D., "NCHS Data Brief," no. 327
     (Dec. 2018) US Department of Health and Human Services, 2015–2017.
14 Charlotte Skovlund et. al., "Association of Hormonal Contraception with
     Depression," *JAMA Psychiatry* 73, no. 11 (Nov. 2016), 1154–1162.

Uterine Ablation for Menopause

The treatment involves destroying or ablating the endometrial lining. It is performed in women who have excessive bleeding, typically caused by hormonal imbalance. After ablation, the patient will no longer have menstrual cycles. This treatment is only for women who are done with childbearing. However, it is not a reliable procedure for birth control, because conception, although unlikely, is still possible. It is, however, a great option for women dealing with abnormal bleeding in the perimenopausal period.

Hysterectomy

I'm appalled by the number of women in my office who were told they needed hysterectomies when in actuality, balancing hormones, specifically progesterone, could have carried them through this time. Remember that as we age, we do not ovulate, and therefore do not counterbalance the estrogen with our own natural progesterone produced by the corpus luteum. The effects of estrogen dominance can be easily counterbalanced with natural progesterone. However, if there are structural changes to the uterus, including fibroids and adenomyosis, natural progesterone will not typically be effective in controlling abnormal bleeding.

Even if the physician removes the uterus and leaves the ovaries, the patient now has compromised blood supply to the ovaries, because at least one-third of that blood supply came from the uterus. This does not put them into surgical menopause, but it does affect the ovarian function.

In our current medical model, there is less incentive to offer conservative therapy and counseling, and more incentive to perform procedures. The reality of our healthcare system is that high-volume and/or high-procedure rates are reimbursed at a higher rate than is time spent offering preventative therapy. From a provider standpoint, it doesn't pay to practice preventative medicine. If your doctor is saying you need a hysterectomy due to vaginal bleeding, especially in the absence of large fibroids, then do your research and consider getting a second opinion.

Hormone Pellets

Hormone pellets are quite popular these days, so I want to take a moment to discuss them further. Pellets require a practitioner to make a small incision in your buttocks, into which they insert a hormone pellet every three to six months. That pellet, which can have different hormones, including but not limited to estrogen and testosterone, delivers those hormones to you in a bolus (large dose) before they slowly start to decline. Pellets are designed to slowly deliver hormones throughout this period.

Some women report feeling especially great on pellets, especially in the first month or so. The problem with pellets, however, is that they may cause the blood levels of estrogen or testosterone to rise up into the supraphysiological (significantly above normal) levels before declining. Women like them because they're convenient, but unfortunately, they may be getting extra-high doses of hormones. With these heightened levels of hormones, there can be some unwelcomed side effects.

***

It's important to remember that all of the hormones we've discussed in this chapter are working in concert with one another, and with other organs of the body, such as the thyroid. This is why having an integrative approach to your health and wellness can benefit you. For example, my patient Samantha came in about a year after her initial visit; at this point, she was well informed about hormones and thought she had a grip on them. She had been doing better, but she reported feeling like she had recently returned to that dark emotional space she had been in when we first met. She wrote me an email and said, "I think I need more progesterone. I can't sleep, and I'm very irritable. Can you increase my progesterone dose?" As reasonable as her request was, I knew that hormones can be super tricky, and I needed to evaluate the whole picture.

She came into the office, and we did her labs. It turned out that her thyroid was completely off, due to her coexisting Hashimoto's disease. Because her life had calmed down, her Hashimoto's disease was not as active as it had been. As a result, her thyroid dose needed to be lowered. Too much thyroid hormone can mimic too little progesterone, with sleep disruption and irritability. She didn't need progesterone; what she needed was to lower her thyroid dose. Sure enough, within just a few days on a lower thyroid dose, she was feeling better. Her case is a perfect example of a patient not recognizing the significant overlap and fluctuations of hormones and their relation to other conditions.

For this reason, it's important for your practitioner to take the time to listen to you and your symptoms. There is no one-size-fits-all in terms of hormone treatment, and everybody is different. It can take a practitioner months of tweaking until the perfect hormone preparation is determined. Whether you choose to take hormones or not, the perimenopausal and menopausal years are a great time to start being reflective about your stressors, your thoughts, your diet, your drinking, and your relationships. As we will discuss fully in the following chapters, health and wellness will never be found in one pill. It's a lifestyle, and adopting it as one, and revering it as one, can lead you down a path of balance and wholeness.

CLOSING TAKEAWAYS

1. Measuring hormones is not as important as evaluating the symptoms that accompany perimenopause. One of the best ways to evaluate your hormone levels is through a twenty-four-hour urine collection because it collects the total amount of hormones over a full day, as opposed to getting a spot evaluation of your hormones through blood testing.

2. If you're going to replace a hormone, it makes sense to replace it as closely to the one that your body already produces. There are multiple FDA-approved bioidentical hormones on the market. Bioidentical hormones are no safer than synthetic hormones.

3. If you are considering HRT, you should weigh the consequences and compare quality-of-life versus potential side effects and start within ten years of menopause and before sixty years of age.

4. There is no right or wrong when deciding about HRT. If you do not have absolute contraindications to HRT, you should weigh risk/benefit and make an informed decision with a provider versed in HRT.

CHAPTER 5

WHY AM I SO TIRED?! UNDERSTANDING THE THYROID/ADRENAL CONNECTION

Andrea presented at age fifty with a strong family history of autoimmune disorders, and was herself diagnosed with discoid lupus in her early twenties. When we met, she was a recently divorced, single mom to three children and working full time as an attorney. She suspected her thyroid was abnormal, for good reason: both her father and mother had severe forms of disease affecting their brain and kidneys. She had already endured years of fatigue, hair loss, and intolerance to cold. Losing weight seemed impossible, and focusing on detailed projects was getting more difficult.

She presented as so many women do with thyroid issues. She had visited multiple doctors over the years who assured her that her thyroid was normal. When I reviewed her labs, however, they were nowhere close to normal, even by conventional criteria. In addition to her abnormal thyroid levels, she had autoantibodies attacking her thyroid, a condition known as Hashimoto's disease. This was not surprising, considering her personal and family history of autoimmune disease. I promptly started her on thyroid replacement and educated her on the importance of lifestyle and diet. Three months later, she returned a new woman. She was starting to lose the stubborn weight and maintained enough energy to exercise and focus.

I wish I could say that this was an uncommon experience, but unfortunately it's not. Because of my own experiences and those of my patients who have suffered unnecessarily, I'm hypervigilant in seeking the potential hormonal etiology in patients suffering with fatigue and depression. Of course, hypothyroidism is not the cause in many cases, but when we are able to find it, it is gratifying to change a life by diagnosing this common disorder.

When you don't have a good, functioning thyroid, life really sucks. Sometimes, I think back to all the years I missed because I had an undiagnosed thyroid disease. I struggled with fatigue, infertility, and depression—all common symptom of thyroid disorders. So much of what I suffered from had so much to do with my hormones and thyroid. Even as a doctor, I couldn't help myself, because I wasn't informed. This is why it is my goal to educate and validate women to be unsilenced advocates for their own health. Don't lose years, relationships, or families because of your health. Do your research and find practitioners who listen and are willing to delve deeper into the root cause of your issue. I decided to devote an entire chapter to thyroid health because declining thyroid function is one of the major issues that I see in my practice every day—and one that I have personally experienced. There are many myths and much misinformation surrounding thyroid health, so read on to learn the realities of this often-undiagnosed issue.

THE THYROID CONVERSATION

When a woman presents with the same symptoms that robbed me of ten years of my life, I look closely at her thyroid. I don't want my patients to lose years of their lives, as I did.

In discussing the number of cases of undiagnosed thyroid disorders, bestselling author and functional health doctor Amy Myers boldly asserts, "In my opinion, [overlooking a diagnosis] is close to medical malpractice. Anyone male or female should automatically be given a complete thyroid panel if they are complaining of any of the thyroid symptoms."[15] I completely agree with this. (For a list of suggested readings on thyroid health, please the Resources section.)

Because of my personal experience with the debilitating effects of thyroid dysfunction, how I treat the thyroid is different from what I learned in medical school. I had to learn from experience and develop alternative and integrative treatments. Even with my own personal experience taking compounded T3, for example, I was

> **If not for my personal experiences, I'm confident that I would still be practicing medicine the way I was trained—and missing the diagnoses of hundreds of women walking through the doors of my practice.**

nervous about stepping out of the traditional box. I worried whether this was safe medicine, and what my "conventional medicine" colleagues would think. If not for my personal experiences, I'm confident that I would still be practicing medicine the way I was trained—and missing the diagnoses of hundreds of women walking

---

15 Amy Myers, *The Thyroid Connection: Why You Feel Tired, Brain-Fogged, and Over-weight—and How to Get Your Life Back* (New York: Little, Brown and Company, 2016), 49.

through the doors of my practice.

Often when I tell patients that I suspect their thyroid is causing their symptoms, they respond, "But my doc said my thyroid levels were normal!" I refrain from rolling my eyes each time I hear this because I know that at least 25 percent of the time women are told their levels are normal despite an actual underlying issue. But their levels are *not* normal, at least not the levels that matter.

Thyroid issues are one of the most under-diagnosed and life-altering conditions. I have many patients who have suffered for years; and it's not their fault. If you go to a doctor and the doctor tells you things are normal, then you accept that things are normal. Do your own research, know the symptoms to look for, and acknowledge if you experience them. If the symptoms persist, listen to your body and follow up, maybe with a different doctor who won't take "normal" for a definitive diagnosis. This can be challenging because we are conditioned to listen to and respect what the doctor tells us. But an important part of maturation and menopause is finding your voice and trusting what your body is saying.

Medical Deep Dive

The thyroid is a gland in the neck, located below the Adam's apple, responsible for metabolic function of cells. It's your motor. When it is inactive, your energy, mood, and motivation are sluggish. Nothing is good when your thyroid is bad. Its job is to secrete thyroid hormones, which have systemic effects on the body.

The output of these hormones is regulated by thyroid-stimulating hormone (TSH), which is produced by the anterior pituitary gland in response to blood levels of thyroid hormone. The lower the circulating thyroid hormone, the higher the TSH. The anterior pituitary is like a thermostat. When you have low levels of thyroid, then the anterior pituitary secretes more TSH, which stimulates the thyroid to create more thyroid hormone. Conversely, when you have high levels of thyroid hormone, the anterior pituitary stops producing thyroid.

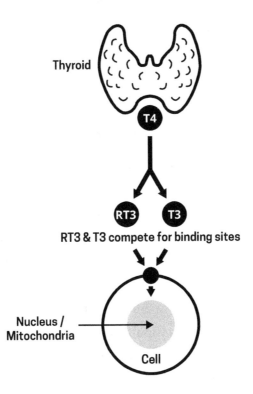

How the Thyroid Works

TSH causes the thyroid to make thyroxine (T4), which has to be converted into triiodothyronine (T3). T3 is the active form and is what actually affects the cell. There is a lot of contradictory information in the field of thyroid health, but one point that is not debatable is that you need to have active T3.

MYTH

Medical providers all use the same criteria to evaluate thyroid status.

REALITY

There is a great deal of debate about which thyroid lab values to consider in the diagnosis of hypothyroidism.

You can discern much about your thyroid health without being a doctor. It's true that things can get pretty complicated when it comes to treating the thyroid, but anyone can start to do their own research to dispel the common myths around thyroid testing. Start by getting your blood drawn using the following labs listed. Comprehensive labs are an essential part of your thyroid health assessment. Many providers will only draw TSH. However, in order to gain a comprehensive view of thyroid function, other labs should be obtained. Ask your doctor for the following comprehensive thyroid analysis to achieve a complete understanding of your thyroid's functionality.

THYROID HORMONE LABS TO OBTAIN

- TSH

- Free T4—Free-circulating thyroid hormone not bound to blood proteins

- Free T3—Free-circulating active thyroid hormone unbound to blood proteins

- Reverse T3—Inactive thyroid hormone

- Thyroid peroxidase antibodies (TPO)—Autoantibodies present that attack thyroid tissue. The most common antibodies identified in Hashimoto's disease

- Thyroglobulin antibodies—Autoantibodies present that attack thyroid tissue and the second most common antibodies identified in Hashimoto's disease

Interpreting thyroid labs can be tricky. Doctors have relied on TSH testing to help diagnose and treat patients with a thyroid disorder, but the problem with understanding thyroid health is that there is no consensus on what values thyroid hormones must be, especially TSH. Practitioners of conventional medicine believe the myth that the most important lab to consider is TSH, and if your TSH is in a certain level, then you're "normal." This is why your doctor might tell you your thyroid levels are normal, even though your symptoms remain. Optimal TSH value is between 1.5 and 2.0 (values between 2.0 and 3.0 may represent a problem; above 3.0 should be considered abnormal).

Furthermore, it is likely that just looking at a laboratory value like TSH, while useful, is not the only data that should be relied upon. History, physical exam, and other lab tests can be very important in helping to establish what is optimal for the individual. Doctors sometimes forget that the treatment should be individualized to each patient, rather than putting everyone in the same box.

I cannot stress enough how important it is to ALWAYS get a personal copy of your labs either directly from your practitioner, the patient portal, or the lab directly. It's essential to look at all of the labs described above. Conventionally practicing providers will use stricter criteria to make the diagnosis of hypothyroidism. Know your numbers! Solving the thyroid mystery can be life changing.

SYMPTOMS OF HYPOTHYROIDISM

- Feeling tired, weak, or depressed
- Dry skin or brittle nails
- Constipation
- Cold intolerance
- Memory problems
- Difficulty thinking clearly
- Heavy or irregular menstrual periods
- Weight gain
- Infertility
- Neck goiter
- Hair loss
- Slow heart rate
- Less sweating than usual
- A puffy face
- A hoarse voice

SYMPTOMS OF HYPERTHYROIDISM (MUCH LESS COMMONLY DIAGNOSED)

- Anxiety
- Insomnia
- Diarrhea
- Weight loss
- High blood pressure
- Rapid heart rate
- Eye sensitivity/bulging
- Vision changes

The Thyroid and Other Conditions

Certain autoimmune diseases, like Hashimoto's thyroiditis and even celiac disease, can disrupt the thyroid. The majority of people with an autoimmune disorder related to the thyroid will have the thyroid peroxidase antibodies (TPO). Nevertheless, there is a subset of patients, like myself, who don't have TPO antibodies. I was testing myself for Hashimoto's disease because I have other autoimmune diseases, and where there is one autoimmune disease, there are likely others; when I looked at my TPO, however, I didn't have any TPO antibodies. After careful research, I learned about thyroglobulin antibodies. When I tested for those, I had them. Eureka! I now apply my personal experience to my patients. If a patient presents without antibodies, but I know they have an autoimmune disease, then I'll look for more thyroid antibodies.

Understanding thyroid dysfunction's relation to autoimmunity is imperative, as there are several dietary and lifestyle factors that influence thyroid function over time. We will talk in later chapters about the role that diet, inflammation, and lifestyle play in your health, but for now, let me mention stress as it relates to thyroid function. When your stress level is high, you convert more of your T4 into reverse T3, as opposed to free T3. That conversion suppresses your metabolism. When you have elevated cortisol levels, it negatively impacts the hypothalamus pituitary loop. The higher the levels of the cortisol, the slower your thyroid production. Therefore, when you're stressed, your body signals your thyroid to work less optimally and it doesn't allow for you to convert free T3, the necessary type of thyroid hormone that you need. Furthermore, if you've had infection, radiation, trauma, even exposure to fluoride or toxins such as mercury and lead, your thyroid function may be disrupted.

Once you have been given a diagnosis, taking thyroid hormone isn't always the answer. Sometimes, I'll have a patient who has border-line thyroid function and isn't incapacitated by it, but isn't functioning optimally either. Just by giving her a supplement that focuses on thyroid health, she will notice an improvement in how she is feeling. Please see the Resources section for further suggestions on thyroid-related materials.

Thyroid Treatments

Once you know your thyroid levels using the lab tests listed, make sure that you find a doctor who will listen to you, because, unfortunately, there are many who won't. If that is the case, then move on until you find a physician who will. You might want to look for integrative physicians or naturopaths in your area to facilitate your thyroid treatment and care. As you can see in the following box, there are many lifestyle and diet changes you can make today that will greatly benefit your thyroid functioning tomorrow.

LIFESTYLE STRATEGIES FOR THYROID SUPPORT
- Repair the gut
- Eliminate gluten and dairy
- Exercise
- HeartMath
- Yoga
- Proper sleep

NUTRITION/SUPPLEMENTS FOR THYROID SUPPORT
- Iron
- Iodine
- Zinc
- Selenium
- Vitamin D

Here's another tricky thing about the thyroid: after the age of fifty, thyroid function starts to decline. Furthermore, the symptoms of low thyroid really overlap with perimenopause. So it can be confusing, even for the doctor. This is why it's so important to be accountable to yourself and understand that if you believe you have a health issue, you must do the work and the research. You must separate the myths from the realities. If you show up at your doctor's office armed with knowledge and insight, then you are more likely to be taken seriously and to get an answer.

WHAT'S UP WITH ADRENALS?

When we talk about menopause and the stages leading up to it, the first hormone that comes to mind is estrogen. And one of the first questions patients ask is, "Do I need hormone replacement therapy?" But what is equally—if not more—important to consider are your adrenal glands.

MYTH

Symptoms of menopause are only related to hormone balance, specifically levels of estrogen.

REALITY

Many of the symptoms of menopause are overactive adrenal function (release of epinephrine/adrenaline), declining thyroid function, and undiagnosed food sensitivities.

The adrenal glands are small walnut-sized glands found on top of your kidneys. There are almost fifty hormones secreted by the adrenals. Approximately 40 percent of sex hormones are secreted by the adrenals in both men and women. This percentage increases as we age. The adrenals are responsible for regulating stress response by secreting two hormones, epinephrine (adrenaline) and norepinephrine (noradrenaline). These hormones act together to prepare us for what has been described as the "fight or flight" response. When they are secreted, heart rate increases, and blood is shunted *toward* essential organs such as the brain and muscles and *away* from the gut and nonessential functions. Blood sugar also rises, due to the conversion of glycogen to glucose.

The problem with stress, from a hormonal perspective, is that your body doesn't differentiate between running late in traffic, finding a rattlesnake in your garage, or a heated confrontation with your beloved. When this sympathetic response is prolonged, it leads to elevated glucose levels and inflammation. Prolonged elevations in cortisol led to elevated blood sugar and metabolic syndrome.

How does this relate to symptoms of menopause? Although the myth is that decreasing estrogen levels alone cause many of the symptoms of menopause, there are several other factors involved. In fact, when hormone levels are measured in perimenopausal women, we frequently see elevated levels of estrogen. This shows that, in reality, the symptoms of menopause are caused by a variety of factors, not just the decreasing levels of one particular hormone. Fluctuations in blood sugar can be as problematic as fluctuations in sex hormones.

Medical Deep Dive

Cortisol is released from the adrenal gland and causes glycogen to be released from the liver. Glycogen breaks down to glucose to provide energy. Short, small doses of cortisol are great and give us the energy boost we need when necessary. But the body is not designed to be under the long-term effects of cortisol. In fact, prolonged cortisol can start to look a lot like menopause. While the adrenal/sex hormone pathway (seen in the following graphic) is supported, the two other pathways are compromised. The focus turns toward the continued production of cortisol, as opposed to supporting the pathway to make sex hormones. This is why stress really can throw your hormones completely off balance.

ADRENAL SEX HORMONE PATHWAY

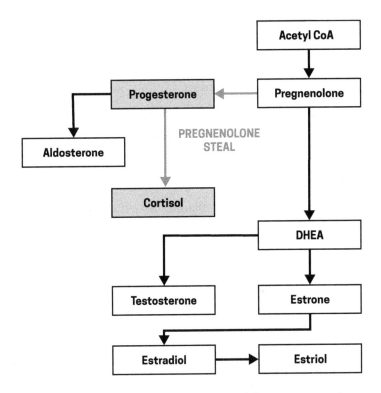

Cortisol is produced as response to stress. If there is an excessive prolonged stress, then pregnenolone is stolen away from producing DHEA and the entire hormonal balance can be upset.

Never underestimate the significance of stress in your life. Even though as medical professionals it's not always easy to draw a straight line from a stressful event to a health crisis, we know that prolonged stress has significant health implications. Stress is like a pebble thrown in water. Its ripple effects can alter our minds, bodies, and emotions. It can impact our families, our work, and our overall health. It is not surprising that there is a correlation between people who are chronically stressed and disease. Adding a poor diet and/or an inflammatory lifestyle, which we'll discuss further in chapter 6, further exacerbates the body's inflammation levels, thus making it more susceptible to illness. The more stress we have, the less ability we have to fight off disease.

CHRONIC STRESS

- Increases abdominal fat
- Impairs cognitive performance
- Suppresses thyroid function
- Creates blood sugar imbalances (hyperglycemia, insulin dys-regulation, metabolic syndrome)
- Causes higher blood pressure
- Decreases bone density and muscle tissue
- Lowers immunity and inflammatory responses

It's pretty easy to imagine the impact stress has on all of our hormones when you consider the fact that the adrenal glands must be supported first. Under stressful scenarios, blood flow is shifted from the gut and kidneys and shifted to the adrenal gland, brain, heart, and muscles. This phenomenon of increasing adrenal output (epinephrine) explains some of the very typical symptoms of anxiety, irritability, insomnia, and sweating.

MYTH

Lack of estrogen is the primary culprit
in menopausal symptoms.

REALITY

The cause of hot flashes is multifactorial. The
most prevalent thinking is that hot flashes
arise as a result of fluctuating estrogen levels.
In actuality, the adrenal gland can secrete norepinephrine and mimic the exact symptoms of
decreased estrogen, hot flashes, and anxiety.

In addressing the symptoms of perimenopause, you must definitely look at the entire concert of hormones. This approach explains
why we need such an extensive evaluation of labs and lifestyle by a
medical provider armed with the realities of menopause and its relationship with other systems.

What's the Deal with Adrenal Fatigue?

After exposure to chronic stress, the adrenal glands may begin to
decrease in its ability to produce cortisol. The reverse side of the coin
creates adrenal fatigue. The term *adrenal fatigue* was coined by Dr.
James Wilson in 1998. In his book *Adrenal Fatigue: The 21st-Century
Stress Syndrome*, he describes a syndrome of fatigue brought on by
chronic stress and/or exposure to certain viruses, including Epstein-
Barr virus (EBV). Most of us are overstimulated and still suffer from
some fatigue.

MYTH

Adrenal fatigue is not a real diagnosis.

REALITY

Chronic stress has serious implications to our health. The medical establishment, however, has been slow to respond to the millions of patients suffering from fatigue/exhaustion. In fact, traditional medical societies, including the Endocrinology Society, assert "no scientific proof exists to support adrenal fatigue as a true medical condition."[16]

Chronic stress increases susceptibility of multiple conditions including:

- Cognitive/memory impairment
- Sleep issues
- Weight gain and blood sugar imbalances
- Heart disease
- Anxiety and depression
- Digestive issues
- Headaches

Of course, other conditions, such as obstructive sleep apnea, diabetes, and thyroid, should be ruled out. In the end, our bodies are not designed to respond to twenty-four-hour stress. Conventional medical providers do not recognize the diagnosis of adrenal fatigue. Whether you believe that adrenal fatigue is a real diagnosis or not, you know more than one or two individuals that are chronically tired.

---

16 "Adrenal Fatigue," Hormone Health Network from the Endocrine Society, accessed March 11, 2019, https://www.hormone.org/diseases-and-conditions/adrenal/adrenal-fatigue.

There is no debate that elevated cortisol levels are deleterious to health. And there is no debate that stress management, proper nutrition, and sleep hygiene mitigate health risks. Please refer to the Resources section for tips/supplements to support adrenal function.

***

As we have noted in this chapter, women's hormones work in concert with one another, which can make diagnoses complicated. Only when a doctor understands this complicated interplay can they effectively treat the systemic health of their patients. An educated patient is an active participant in her own health. In separating thyroid and adrenal myths from reality, it is my hope that you are poised to be a more-engaged contributor to your health diagnoses and treatment plans.

CLOSING TAKEAWAYS

1. Acknowledge your thyroid and adrenal symptoms listed in this chapter.

2. If you have a family history of hypothyroidism, be alert for thyroid dysfunction. If your mother, grandmother, or sister has this condition, then your odds increase.

3. Get your blood drawn using the lab tests listed in this chapter. Educate yourself through research. Remember that TSH above 3.0 indicates deceased thyroid function; and TSH between 2.0 and 3.0 is also concerning.

4. If you have a diagnosis of hypothyroidism, determine if you have Hashimoto's thyroiditis. Understanding

the impact of autoimmunity is critical to your overall health.

5. Find an integrative physician who will listen to you. If there aren't any in your area, look for a naturopath. Unfortunately, even physicians who specialize in hormone disorders (endocrinologist) can underdiagnose disorders of the thyroid and adrenals.

6. Be an Unsilenced Woman—ask questions and speak up. Your health is at stake.

7. The prevalence of thyroid disease and adrenal issues in women is staggering and affects women ten times more frequently than men. This is why it is imperative that you be your own advocate.

CHAPTER 6

FOOD, INFLAMMATION, AND THE GUT: WHAT'S THE GUT GOT TO DO WITH IT?

W hen you are experiencing a health crisis and can't enjoy life the way you want to, you get more inspired to do whatever it takes to feel better, and that often means scrutinizing your life choices and their health effects. Until we systematically look at diet, lifestyle, stressors, gut health, and the realities of our emotional/spiritual states, we are just scratching the surface of our potential health and well-being.

I was diagnosed with lupus in my late twenties. By my thirties, I added the stress of work and family to my already taxed system. I felt worn out and was having a lot of joint pain. I consulted with several traditional doctors, who offered little nutritional advice or support. I knew I needed a different type of doctor who was going to talk to me about diet and lifestyle, because nothing else was working for me. I found my godsend in a doctor that was trained in conventional, integrative, and functional medicine.

In many ways, seeing this doctor changed my life personally and professionally. She explained to me about functional medicine, which looks at the root cause of disease. Rather than prescribe me medications, like my other doctors had advised, this doctor talked at length about diet.

I won't lie—the process of changing my relationship with food was hard, but it was also invaluable. After seeing how much a cleaner diet helped my autoimmune conditions and menopausal symptoms, I became devoted to offering the same knowledge to my patients. In 2009, I entered the integrative medicine fellowship at the University of Arizona. Once I finished my fellowship in integrative medicine, it became important to me to offer a practice that incorporates both functional and integrative approaches. That was the beginning of my practice, Tula Wellness and Aesthetics.

In my practice, we integrate different types of medical specialties and take mind, body, and spiritual approaches to health. We look at the lifestyle, diets, and stress levels of my patients. This field of medicine incorporates all different modalities in order for patients to heal themselves. The underlying motive for this type of health practice is to honor the innate ability the body has to heal itself when provided with the proper nutrition and a healthy lifestyle. The catalyst for this healing transformation starts with a Food Elimination Diet. We will get into the specifics of this life-changing, habit-breaking diet, but first let's discuss some of the effects that food has on the body.

THE EFFECTS OF FOOD ON OUR HEALTH

We know which foods are good for us and which aren't, and yet we invariably consume foods each day that make us feel sluggish and inflamed. When is it going to stop? When you know something is going to make you feel bad, when you know there's nothing to gain from eating this ice cream, for example, but you eat it anyway—that's an addiction. Unless you've taken steps to clean up your diet, you may not realize the subtle ways that your food is making you sick. You might be surviving, but you're not feeling, looking, or being your best.

> Unless you've taken steps to clean up your diet, you may not realize the subtle ways that your food is making you sick.

In David A. Kessler's *The End of Overeating: Taking Control of the Insatiable American Appetite,* he exposes the ugly truth that our food is engineered to be addictive: "There's still a lot we don't know about the relationship between the dopamine-driven motivational system and our behavior in the presence of rewarding foods. But we do know that foods high in sugar, fat, and salt are altering the biological circuitry of our brains."[17] Kessler goes on to assert that when you combine salt, sugar, and fat in certain combinations, it stimulates the same centers in the brain as nicotine or crack cocaine. Think about that. When potato chip companies say, "You can't eat just one," they are being literal, and its engineered that way on purpose! When comparing brain scans after eating a potato chip with scans after consuming crack cocaine, the same areas are lit up in the brain and the same endorphins are released.

---

17   David A. Kessler, *The End of Overeating: Taking Control of the Insatiable American Appetite* (New York: Rodale, 2009), 60.

We rarely discuss the seriousness of our cultural food addiction, but part of why so many people feel bad is because of the daily choices we make surrounding food. (For more information, including a list of documentaries about food production in our culture, please see the Resources section.) Many Americans would rather take a pill than address their food addiction. We want the easy solution, but there is no easy solution when it comes to food.

Unfortunately, most communities don't make it easy for you to make the healthiest food choices. It's much easier, faster, and cheaper to get a burger and fries in most communities than it is to get an acai bowl. If you take your relationship to food seriously, and understand it as a true addiction, then you understand that you have to retrain your brain and your taste buds. Even the healthiest gurus have to make decisions each day about what they consume. I find that even though I know eating certain foods makes me feel uncomfortable, my brain overrides that logic, and sometimes I eat them anyway.

What Does Food Have to Do with Menopause and Hormones?

Some of my healthiest patients who have breezed through menopause have one thing in common: they have embraced a plant-based diet and essentially eliminated inflammatory foods, such as animal fats and dairy. The average patient, however, is not ready or even willing to make such an immediate adjustment. Even so, removing these food triggers is one of the most effective ways to feel your best throughout peri/menopause. If you're not ready to make that leap, then I would encourage you to start with some basic principles listed in this chapter.

You can take all the supplements and hormone replacement therapy you want, but if you're not paying attention to the food you consume, then you're never going to feel your best. Part of that has to do with our gut and its permeability. Hormone health is directly related to gut health, and it's even more directly related to how you're going to feel throughout the peri/menopausal years.

I have put many of my patients on a Food Elimination Diet and for the vast majority of them, their symptoms improved. The hard part about food is that when you're going

> You can take all the supplements and hormone replacement therapy you want, but if you're not paying attention to the food you consume, then you're never going to feel your best.

through perimenopause, you're not feeling well. You might feel tired, or you might feel sluggish, so you reach for a cookie. You feel happy for about ten minutes. Then that cookie makes you feel sluggish and tired, so you reach for another. It's a constant cycle of trying to feel better, but you keep reaching for the things that make you feel badly. Hello, addiction.

These are difficult alterations to make because we're attached to food culturally and socially. So much of what we experience is centered on food. I grew up eating eggs, grits, and bacon and that was considered a *good* breakfast. I had no idea of how inflammatory and toxic that diet was.

Food Allergies, Sensitivities, and Intolerances

My personal experience with food sensitivities is the reason I prescribe the Food Elimination Diet to just about every patient who walks through the door. You can't possibly know how good you can feel until you do this diet; I'm absolutely convinced of it. Until you take out all potential trigger foods, you have no idea how bad you're feeling as a result of eating certain foods.

You may think that getting tested for food allergies is the best way to determine your sensitivities. These tests can be helpful, but they do not take the place of removing the common food triggers. There are many tests out there, but you have to understand there's a difference between a food allergy and a food sensitivity. Many of these subtle sensitivities may not show up on a blood test, but that doesn't mean that your body isn't undergoing a physical, systemic response to the food trigger. One of the best ways to determine what foods you're sensitive to is to eliminate the foods and then add them back in slowly through a Food Elimination Diet.

It doesn't really matter if I test somebody and I tell them, "You're sensitive to corn." A better teaching method is for you to see how you feel without corn in your diet. You're being *shown* the problem rather than being *told* the problem, which is a powerful distinction. Furthermore, just because the lab test says you have a sensitivity, that doesn't necessarily tell you how it affects your everyday life—like headaches, fatigue, fuzzy thinking. For example, I love tomatoes, but during my own Food Elimination Diet, I realized that they cause me headaches, fatigue, and joint pain. Tomatoes are nightshades, and individuals with autoimmune disorders are particularly sensitive to this class of food. For me, the only reason I'm able to continue to avoid tomatoes is because I know how good I can feel without eating them.

Typical food sensitivity symptoms include headaches and joint pain. In fact, I've successfully treated 90 percent of my patients with migraines through a Food Elimination Diet. Headaches are traditionally caused by certain trigger foods. But those triggers are different for each person, which is why it is important to learn what your own triggers are, as well as your responses to those triggers. For example, I'm not allergic to gluten. If I took a blood test, it would not show any allergy to gluten. It may not even show up as a sensitivity. However, because I've done an elimination diet, I know that when I eat gluten, I feel depressed and have cloudy thinking. Nobody ever told me that bread affects how well my brain functions, but I know it to be true for my body.

Many of us have food sensitivities of some sort. The reactions to these foods are not the lips-swelling-skin-rash kind of response. It's subtle. It's insidious. I wasn't sick, but eating gluten every day changed my quality of life. I would go through each day exhausted and with a sluggish mind.

Food Allergy, Sensitivity, and Intolerance:

- *Food allergy* is when you eat a food and have a physical response, like your lips start to swell or your throat starts to close. You can't eat that food. You have to be prepared to take Benadryl or epinephrine. It can be life-threatening in certain circumstances.

- *Food sensitivity* is when you eat a certain food and you have a non-life-threatening reaction. It's not an allergic reaction. It's actually an entirely different immune response you're having. There are different types of antibodies that your body creates when you are sensitive to a food.

- *Food intolerance* is another category of food response. An intolerance is similar to a sensitivity, but your body is a little bit more resistant to the offending food. With an intolerance, our body is not able to break down those foods. Lactose intolerance is a good example. Approximately 75 percent of African-Americans, 90 percent of Asians, and 15 percent of Caucasians are lactose intolerant.[18]

---

18 D.L. Swagerty, A.D. Walling, and R.M. Klein, "Lactose Intolerance," *American Family Physician* 65, no. 9 (May 1, 2002), 1845-1850.

You'd be surprised at the food that you might be sensitive to. If you have a thyroid condition or any autoimmune disorder, for example, you might be particularly sensitive to nightshades, legumes, and grains in general. Another important point to remember is that as we age, we tend to become more sensitive to food. So, foods that you could eat as a teenager may now cause bloating, fatigue, and other symptoms. We typically don't associate symptoms like exhaustion and brain fog with what we ate the day before, but we must pay attention to the foods we consume and their effects, no matter how subtle. Furthermore, our food is continuing to be modified and changed in ways that our bodies don't even recognize. The best way to be an advocate for your own health and vitality is to make smart, intentional decisions about the foods you consume to reduce inflammation and disease in your body.

> Gut health, like inflammation, is at the core of just about every disease there is. Even so, the gut is one of the most neglected organs in the body.

Gut Health

The cure to many health issues and menopausal symptoms starts in the gut. Gut health, like inflammation, is at the core of just about every disease there is. Even so, the gut is one of the most neglected organs in the body. It's more involved in our immunity and our nervous system than any other organ, even our brain. This important correlation is not taught to doctors or patients. There's a big misunderstanding—or really miseducation—of how important the gut is. The myth is that gut health only affects your gastro-intestinal system; the reality, however, is that the gut has systemic effects on all systems of our bodies. The gut is full of bacteria and too much of any good thing can be a bad thing. Just as our hormones need to be in balance, so does our gut flora.

MYTH

Gut health only relates to gastro-intestinal health.

REALITY

The gut affects multiple systems in the body, particularly immunity and nervous system function. More and more research is proving that the more permeable our gut is, the more impacted we are by the foods that we're eating.

Gut health starts with what we put in our mouths because food affects the permeability of the intestinal lining. This intestinal lining must function properly. When it is dysfunctional, we refer to this as *intestinal permeability*, or *leaky gut*. Leaky gut describes a gut that has been damaged. A person with leaky gut does not have the same immune defenses as a person with an impermeable intestinal lining. I'm often asked, "Does leaky gut really exist?" Conventional doctors don't quite understand it and it is not recognized as an official medical condition with an accompanying ICD-10 code. As a medical student, I never heard any mention of leaky gut. You can understand why many doctors and insurance companies still don't consider it an actual disease, but it undoubtedly has far-reaching, systemic effects on the health of our bodies. More and more research is proving that the more permeable our gut is, the more impacted we are by the foods that we're eating. When it comes to gut health, it is, unfortunately, taking a long time for conventional medicine to catch up with new research.

HEALTHY GUT VS. LEAKY GUT

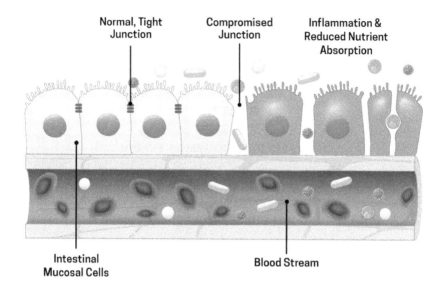

Normal, Tight Junction

Compromised Junction

Inflammation & Reduced Nutrient Absorption

Intestinal Mucosal Cells

Blood Stream

Our gut is designed to be a spherical tube that absorbs nutrients and protects the body from some of the things that we eat. When there's damage to that lining, undigested food particles are able to breach that barrier and get into the bloodstream. The body senses these particles as foreign intruders and essentially attacks them, leading to a response similar to that of an autoimmune disease. This is when our daily choices become so important. It's not only the food we eat, but it's the sleep we get, the stress we feel, even the medicines we take. For example, steroids, antibiotics, and NSAIDS exacerbate a leaky gut.

There are many symptoms that suggest you have a leaky gut. For example, joint pain, difficulty concentrating, inability to lose weight, swelling of joints, and chronic fatigue syndrome. When you mention these symptoms, and the ones listed next, the gut isn't necessarily the first thing that you think about, but these are some of the more obvious signs of leaky gut.

SIGNS AND SYMPTOMS OF LEAKY GUT

- Allergies
- Anxiety
- Autoimmune disease
- Autism
- Bloating
- Chronic fatigue syndrome
- Digestive problems
- Fatigue
- Food sensitivities
- Headaches
- Inflammatory bowel disease
- Irritable bowel syndrome
- Inflammatory skin conditions
- Joint pain
- Mood issues and autism
- Syndrome X
- Thyroid conditions
- Weight gain

Research is showing that many autoimmune conditions are associated with leaky gut, as well as neurological and neurodegenerative diseases, such as Parkinson's and Alzheimer's. Almost all diseases can be linked back to inflammation, and thereby a leaky gut. Furthermore, your hormones are directly affected by your gut health. Metabolizing hormones, especially estrogen, is important in the gut. If you are constipated, for example, you are not excreting excess estrogen. Without proper gut health, you don't have proper bowel function, which causes a backflow of hormones to be re-released back into your body. This could lead to symptoms of estrogen dominance.

TREATMENT FOR LEAKY GUT

Luckily the gut can be repaired, though it takes time, discipline, and patience. The most effective treatment for leaky gut is the 4R Program.

Leaky Gut 4R Program:
1. Remove
2. Restore
3. Repair
4. Reinoculate

The first step is to *remove* the food that is taxing your gut by following the Food Elimination Diet described in detail at the end of this chapter. The next step is to *restore* the gut, which entails giving back to the body things that are required for food digestion. Stomachs need the proper pH in order to digest food. Not having that proper pH or enough hydrochloric acid in the stomach can cause problems, such as heartburn. Food has to be broken down so it can be absorbed. The body uses digestive enzymes to accomplish this. We use certain digestive enzymes to break down milk; we use others located in the bile to break down fat. Some enzymes, like hydrochloric acid, are needed to break down all foods. Pancreatic enzymes are important because they break down plants, fat, and many other foods. Sometimes we need to take supplements to restore this part of the digestive process. If you are having symptoms such as nausea, abdominal discomfort, or heartburn immediately after eating, you might benefit from restoring your gut with digestive enzymes, bile acids, or hydrochloric acid.

The next step to treating a leaky gut is to begin *repairing* the intestinal wall. We can do that with supplements and healing foods, like bone broth. Basically at this stage of gut repair, we are attempting to reduce the chronic inflammation of the intestinal wall.

Supplements to Repair a Leaky Gut:

- L-Glutamine
- Vitamin D
- Zinc
- Vitamin A
- Aloe vera
- Omega-3 fatty acids

It is happening slowly, but doctors are gaining more understanding and awareness of the importance of gut health, especially the bacteria of the gut. In the final phase of treating a leaky gut, we *reinoculate* the gut with healthy bacteria, called prebiotics and probiotics. Prebiotic foods promote the growth of beneficial bacteria in the intestines, whereas the probiotic is the bacteria itself. The prebiotic acts as fuel for the probiotics to work more effectively. Both are important in gut function, and sources of both are listed below. The addition of fermented foods such as sauerkraut, kimchi, miso, yogurt, kefir, and kombucha is also important in restoring the bacterial balance.

Common Probiotics for Gut Health:

- Lactobacillus
- Bifidobacterium
- Saccharomyces boulardii (a yeast)

Fermented Foods:

- Sauerkraut
- Kimchi
- Yogurt—unsweetened
- Kombucha
- Natto
- Kefir

- Raw cheese
- Apple cider vinegar
- Tempe
- Miso
- Kvass

Prebiotic-Rich Foods:

- Raw chicory root
- Jerusalem artichoke
- Dandelion greens
- Garlic
- Leek
- Onions
- Asparagus
- Banana
- Apples
- Burdock root
- Flax seeds
- Jicama root
- Seaweed

THE INFLAMMATION SITUATION

Mary came to me complaining of feeling bloated and achy most days, as well as experiencing hot flashes, mood swings, and extreme fatigue. As I do with most patients, I placed her on the Food Elimination Diet. I knew that if she discovered her trigger foods and eliminated them, we could decrease inflammation and alleviate a lot of her symptoms without further treatment. In addition to the Food Elimination Diet, I also added four grams of omega-3, and daily doses of vitamin D and turmeric to Mary's diet. One test to objectively measure the body's inflammation level is called C-reactive protein (hsCRP). It's also used as a marker to assess a patient's cardiac risk. I often order this test to help patients get a visual—a number—of how inflamed they are. Mary's results showed her CRP level was 9.5 (normal range is 0–2)! I sent her home to complete her Food Elimination Diet and asked that she return in three months. When she returned, she had lost twelve pounds, and her CRP level was down to 3.8. Furthermore, she went from being pre-diabetic to having normal glucose levels.

This is impressive, especially considering this result was achieved without any medication, only the addition of supplements and the elimination of trigger foods. Her results were an overall decrease in her systemic inflammation, and she was pleased to discover her symptoms disappeared without further medical intervention.

Inflammation is a healthy response that under normal circumstances doesn't cause damage to our bodies. A prolonged inflammatory response, however, taxes the immune system and puts us at risk for disease. Inflammation increases blood sugar and impacts thyroid function, cognitive performance, blood pressure, and immune response. Furthermore, inflammation increases the severity and susceptibility to disease and causes the release of what we call *pro-inflammatory cytokines*. Science has shown that if we can break this cycle of inflammation, then we can prevent, and in many cases reverse, disease.

As evidenced by patients like Mary, some of the disturbances of perimenopause and menopause can be remedied by managing the body's inflammation levels. In addition to decreasing hot flashes and weight gain, this shift in daily life can have profound impacts on your body's systemic inflammation levels. This lowers your chances of disease, obesity, and many other chronic conditions. Don't underestimate the power of your daily choices. Food can be your medicine or your poison. When you approach food as a medicine, it changes your perspective and has the power to change your health. Begin making small decisions today that can drastically improve your health tomorrow.

> Don't underestimate the power of your daily choices. Food can be your medicine or your poison. When you approach food as a medicine, it changes your perspective and has the power to change your health.

Diet's Role in Inflammation

Eating foods daily from the following pro-inflammatory foods list creates chronic inflammation in our bodies, and that is exactly what leads to disease. Avoid refined sugars, trans fats, including partially hydrogenated margarine and vegetable shortening, and imbalanced cooking oils.

Conversely there are many foods you can eat to support your body's natural, healthy functioning. Anti-inflammatory foods include healthy fats and vegetables. You want to get a wide variety of vegetables and look for dense and bright colors.

When it comes to fish and seafood, choose wild-caught because farm-raised foods do not contain the nutritional value and the omega-3 content. Also remember that the larger the fish, the higher amount of potential toxins, including mercury. Similarly, when you choose fruit, choose organic. Blueberries, blackberries, and strawberries are considered anti-inflammatory, though not all fruits are, so consult the chart below when choosing your fruits.

Pro-Inflammatory Foods:

- Refined sugars
- Trans fats (partially hydrogenated oils, margarine, vegetable shortening)
- Imbalanced cooking oils (polyunsaturated, safflower, corn, sunflower)
- Processed meats
- Refined grains

Anti-Inflammatory Foods:

- Healthy fats (extra virgin olive oil, expeller pressed canola)
- Vegetables (eat all the colors of the rainbow)
- Fish and seafood (salmon, black cod)
- Fruit (organic, berries)
- Beans, legumes, and pasta (cooked al dente)
- Whole and cracked grains
- Cooked Asian mushrooms
- Red wine
- Tea (white, green, oolong)
- Dark chocolate (with at least 70 percent cocoa)
- Supplements (omega-3 fatty acids)

Tips for Anti-Inflammatory Food Health

OMEGA-3 VERSUS OMEGA-6

When it comes to fats, we want a good balance. The typical American diet is high in omega-6 and low in omega-3; this diet is associated with an increase in cytokines and all the proteins that are released from cells that trigger inflammation. Healthy fats include extra-virgin olive oil, walnuts, avocados, hemp, and flaxseeds.

FIBER

Fiber helps reduce the transit time of food through your gut. If you're eating a processed food, and you combine that with fiber, then you have, in some ways, diminished the impact of eating the processed food. Fiber slows the absorption of food and subsequently reduces the sharp fluctuations in blood sugar. A good example of this difference is seen in instant oatmeal versus steel-cut oats. If you are eating instant oatmeal and just pouring hot water, that oatmeal has already been processed. Your body doesn't have to do any work, so you're not getting the nutritional value that you're getting from steel-cut oats.

Generally speaking, the more processed a food, the more inflammatory it will be. Conversely, the more our bodies have to work in order to digest and break down food, the better it is for us. For example, if you cook a whole-wheat pasta to the point where you can't recognize it's a noodle, then you're not going to get the same benefit as you would a pasta that was cooked al dente. Similarly, when selecting grains and breads, remember that the higher the fiber and the less processed the bread or grain is, the better it is for you.

WHAT ABOUT WINE?

Red wine is one of the anti-inflammatory foods that people often misuse. The good news is that small amounts of red wine are considered anti-inflammatory. The detail to remember here, is *small amounts,* meaning four to six ounces. Keep in mind that a *serving* of wine is not the same as a *glass* of wine. Often when patients say, "Oh, I have two glasses of wine a night," they're probably drinking closer to four to six glasses based on what the average pour is at home. It often triggers hot flashes and disrupted sleep for many women. Be mindful of this when drinking wine. It might benefit you to cut it out altogether. (Please don't send me hate mail!)

For many women, the act or ritual of drinking wine is as satisfying as the drink itself. If you are having difficulty eliminating wine, consider creating what I call a "mindful drinking experience." First, find the smallest wine glass you have. Then open the bottle mindfully and pour your designated amount (four to six ounces). Take a moment to smell the wine, to swirl it around your glass. Take small sips if you want your wine to last through dinner, or your bath, or whatever your ritual is. I often find it's not the alcohol itself that is relaxing people; it's the ritual surrounding it. If you find that one serving of wine isn't enough for you, try adding in a second serving of another drink, like sparkling water with lime.

TEA

Another drink option to help combat inflammation is tea—white tea, green tea, and oolong tea. An excellent tea choice that is high in antioxidants is matcha tea. Matcha tea is a powdered tea made from plants that are shaded and harvested in a special way. When you drink matcha tea, you're actually drinking the tea leaves themselves. Matcha also has more antioxidants than a regular cup of steeped green tea. It also has a slower release of caffeine, so it gives you more clarity and energy, and it's also great for metabolizing blood sugar.

NUTRIENT-DENSE FOODS

For an anti-inflammatory diet, try to include as many servings of the nutrient-dense foods listed below as possible. These are the foods packed with vitamins and minerals and are healthy ways to support your body's natural balance.

Nutrient-Dense Foods:
- Kale, watercress
- Collard greens
- Bok choy

- Spinach
- Brussels sprouts
- Swiss chard
- Arugula
- Radish
- Cabbage
- Bean sprouts

The foods listed above are considered superfoods because of their nutrient-dense composition. There are many ways that you can ingest these foods, so if you don't like eating them, you can easily add them to smoothies or juices. Try to consume several servings of superfoods each week. Kale, in particular, is a cruciferous vegetable, and like other vegetables in this category—like broccoli and brussels sprouts—it contains hormone-balancing qualities. Other foods that can also help create and maintain hormone equilibrium are listed below. Each of these can aid your body during the years of peri/menopause.

Hormone-Balancing Foods:
- Maca
- Raw cacao
- Chia seeds
- Hemp seeds
- Iodine-rich foods like chlorella and sea vegetables

THE FOOD ELIMINATION DIET

In order to address my symptoms of fatigue, headaches, and joint pain, my doctor recommended the Food Elimination Diet for eight weeks. She told me I needed to cut out dairy, sugar, alcohol, gluten, corn, soy, and tomatoes. These restrictions made sense to me, especially gluten, but that doesn't mean it was easy. I reluctantly agreed to restrict these foods, even my beloved tomatoes for two months.

Within two to three weeks, I felt better. In fact, I couldn't remember ever feeling that great in my life. My skin glowed. I woke in the morning with energy, and I didn't feel like I was dragging myself out of bed. I slept better. My thoughts were clearer. I was happier. It really was a life-changing event. I felt so good that I promised myself I would never ever eat bread or the other offending foods again.

> Within two to three weeks, I felt better. In fact, I couldn't remember ever feeling that great in my life.

We underestimate the addictive power of our food choices. People struggle daily with food addictions, and our entire food industry is built around this dependence. By doing a Food Elimination Diet, you will start to understand the addictive relationship you have with food. Give yourself plenty of liquids, rest, and self-love during an elimination diet.

If somebody walked up to you and offered you something to take away your pain, make you glow, give you energy and focus, and make you leaner and happier, you'd jump at the chance. The Food Elimination Diet is that answer, but when I tell my patients that, I'm often met with blank stares and an "anything but that" response. Most people don't want to do the work that's required. Unfortunately, without seriously examining the foods you eat, you will not be able to feel your absolute best.

THE 21-DAY FOOD ELIMINATION DIET PLAN

- Avoid the foods on the "Foods to Remove" list below for at least twenty-one days

- Keep a food journal of foods eaten and any physical or emotional symptoms you experience

- Drink plenty of liquids

- Choose organic foods

- Get plenty of rest

Foods to Remove: - *31 craves*

- Corn ✓
- Dairy ✓
- Eggs ✓
- Gluten Grains ✓
- White Sugar ✓
- Shellfish ✓
- Soy ✓
- Beef ✓
- Pork ✓
- Processed Meats ✓
- Coffee, Tea ✓
- Chocolate ✓
- Alcohol ✓
- Tomatoes ✓

Foods to Eat:

- Fruits—organic when possible
- Healthy Oils
- Lean Meats

- Legumes
- Nuts
- Seeds
- Vegetables
- Non-Gluten Whole Grains

It's important to track what you're eating during your Food Elimination Diet. Write down everything you consume (food and drink), and also write down what else you did that day, including what stressors you experienced: How do you feel? What is your mood like? Write down anything you feel is relevant. Sometimes, you'll see patterns that you wouldn't realize without a detailed log.

During the first week of the diet, you can expect a detox period. During this time, you're essentially withdrawing from the influence of certain addictive foods, like caffeine and sugar. It varies for each person, but usually somewhere between day two and four, you're going to start having some detox symptoms. The symptoms last about two days, and you might feel tired, achy, and/or have a headache. If you're going to start a Food Elimination Diet and you have a poor diet to begin with—like a lot of sugar and/or caffeine—you definitely want to start the diet before a weekend, or during a time when you can be at home and rest during your withdrawal symptoms.

Furthermore, you have to really be ready for this diet. There is no cheating because the only person you're cheating is yourself. If you're not willing to do it, then don't, because you'll be wasting your time. Wait until you are ready.

It Gets Better: The Reintroduction Phase

After you have completed at least twenty-one days on the Food Elimination Diet, you may begin reintroducing foods. It doesn't matter what you choose to add first. I always tell people to eat the one thing you've been wanting to eat, that you feel like you've been "deprived of" during the process, but you have to be strategic and only introduce one food at a time.

After my two months on the Food Elimination Diet, I slowly started to reintroduce the foods that I wanted to eat first—tomatoes. When you reintroduce a food after an elimination diet, you don't just eat a little bit; you bring it back hard. You eat multiple portions of it so that you get the full impact. When I reintroduced tomatoes, I felt fine all day. Then the next morning, I woke up and I felt like a truck had hit me. Every single joint in my body hurt. I had a migraine headache. I couldn't think clearly. I was tired. It was really amazing to me. *No, not the tomatoes!* But I had the proof, and there was no denying what my body was telling me. Tomatoes are not my friends. For people who are prone to lots of headaches, joint pain, and fatigue, like myself, nightshades (like tomatoes) can be problematic.

MYTH

As long as I eat foods that are considered healthy, it won't negatively affect my health.

REALITY

A person's relationship with food and health is as unique as the individual. Just because a food is "healthy" doesn't mean it's good for *your* body. You can still have food sensitivities and allergies to foods that are good for most people. This is why the Food Elimination Diet is so useful in determining what is the best way to feed *your* body.

During the reintroduction phase of the diet, you must pay close attention or you can lose your momentum and wreck the experiment. If you start eating whatever you want and you aren't meticulous about making a note of what you consumed and how it made you feel, then you have undone all the work you put in. Write down the foods you are reintroducing and any symptoms you experience, even if they seem unrelated or don't have anything to do with your digestive system. Remember that foods affect your entire physiology, so it's important to pay attention to your mood, headaches, abdominal pain, joint pain, skin irritation, sleep, even nasal congestion.

GUIDELINES FOR REINTRODUCING FOODS

- Days 1 & 2 of Reintroduction Phase—Choose one food that you miss the most. The order of reintroduction is not critical. Eat a generous amount of that food throughout Day 1 (2–3 average size portions), while continuing to eat the other foods from the Elimination Diet. During that day, and the next (Day 2), record any symptoms in your Food Journal.

- Days 3 & 4 and beyond—If there is no reaction to the food during this two-day period, keep that food in the food plan and reintroduce a second food in the same manner (introduce the food on Day 3 and watch for any symptoms on Days 3 & 4). If no reaction, keep that food in the diet and add the third challenge food, and so on.

- If any food is associated with symptoms, stop eating that food immediately, wait until the symptoms clear, and reintroduce the next food. Retest any foods that give symptoms after testing all of the challenge foods using the same procedure of eating the food one day, followed by a one-day waiting period to note your symptoms.

- Potential reactions include diarrhea or constipation, fatigue, depression, anxiety, gas, bloating and/or abdominal pain, headache, muscle or joint pain, skin irritations, itching or break outs, insomnia, sinus congestion or runny nose.

I understand how confused people are about what to eat. There are so many diet and nutrition plans out there. Most of the research finds the healthiest diets to be as plant-based as possible. As much as you can avoid animal fats and processed sugar, you're probably better off.

Unfortunately, we get a lot of mixed messages from the media. The food industries are big-dollar industries that want consumers to believe that eating their food is good for you. Many of those same industries are funding the government's sources that we use as our guides, like the food pyramid. Those industries affect the "healthy" guidelines for how we're supposed to eat. The people who have the most money have the most ability to influence how people live and eat. For this reason, I would recommend that people get as informed as they can about the food industry so they can begin to discern fact from propaganda. (For more resources on choosing healthy foods, visit the Resources section.) An informed consumer is a healthy consumer.

***

I know firsthand the powerful results that can happen after participating in a Food Elimination Diet. It's not easy, but remember the first several days will be the hardest, and then you will start to feel better each day. You will have more energy and clearer focus. You will find that many of your menopausal symptoms might be more manageable or cease altogether. You might notice some desirable effects like a slimmer waist and clearer skin, but below the surface, one of the most important things about doing this plan is that it reduces the amount of inflammation in your body.

The goal of a Food Elimination Diet is to find out which foods are your medicines and which foods are your poisons. It's different for every person. Even things that are classified as healthy, like tomatoes in my case, are not necessarily something you need to be eating. In addition to finding out more about your food reactions, you are also allowing your gut to detox and heal itself. After a Food Elimination Diet, you will begin to see food in an entirely new way. This shift in perspective has the power to change your health and your life.

CLOSING TAKEAWAYS

1. Until we systematically look at diet, lifestyle, stressors, gut health, and the realities of our emotional/spiritual states, we are just scratching the surface of our potential health and well-being.

2. Removing food triggers from your diet is one of the most effective ways to feel your best throughout peri/menopause.

3. Gut health has systemic effects on all systems of our bodies and is at the core of just about every disease.

4. Inflammation is a healthy response that, under normal circumstances, doesn't cause damage to our bodies. A prolonged inflammatory response, however, taxes the immune system and puts us at risk for disease.

5. By doing a Food Elimination Diet, you will start to understand the addictive relationship you have with food.

CHAPTER 7

HEALTHY, SEXY GLOW

The field of aesthetics is a polarizing one. Many people go to great lengths to hold onto their youthful looks. The idea that women are expected, and even pressured, to maintain a youthful look (perky boobs, flat tummies, and chiseled jawlines) is reminiscent of sexual objectification. This is a cultural problem that has far-reaching effects, and if you are struggling with this paradigm, you're not alone. I operated under this bias for a long time until my own experiences changed that.

My own views about aesthetics profoundly shifted when I began losing my eyebrows because of my thyroid condition. I didn't like what my face looked like without eyebrows. I felt like the whole contour of my face changed. Every day I would carefully draw in my eyebrows only for them to fade away by lunchtime. After spending too much time fretting over whether my eyebrows had "melted," I finally decided to get my eyebrows tattooed. That was the first aesthetic procedure I ever had, and it changed my perspective on the whole industry. This one small act made me so much happier in the morning because I knew I had eyebrows. I was able to start the day cheerier, and that's quite a monumental change! I began to understand that changing small things on the outside can be the catalyst to make big changes on the inside.

My journey into aesthetics was more like a stumble. When I started my practice, I had no interest in offering aesthetics. But after the receptionist (who happened to be an aesthetician) realized that women seemed more interested in the face creams and sunscreens than the supplements we offered in the office, we started to offer facials. Request for facials turned into requests for Botox, fillers, and other services that could help with the changes that women were noticing with age. The name Tula Wellness was upgraded to Tula Wellness and Aesthetics. Every service we provide is a direct answer to the needs of aging women.

I was reluctant at first. Admittedly, I had no idea where Botox or filler was injected, not to mention why anyone would want to put it in their face. However, what became increasingly apparent to me was the observation that what a woman sees in the mirror directly correlates with her health and how she feels about herself.

> What a woman sees in the mirror directly correlates with her health and how she feels about herself.

When a woman sits in the aesthetics chair, she brings with her the myriad concerns she has perhaps harbored for years or decades about her personal appearance. But there is so much more than a physical body in the chair. Beneath the physical woman there is a spirit filled with life's joys, disappointments, heartbreaks, and unanswered questions. In this chapter, I want to share with you the countless lessons I have learned from the women in my aesthetics chair.

Many of my patients struggle with the balance between wanting to look "natural" versus "having work done." Everyone wants to look fabulous, but most of my clients don't want anyone to know that they have put any effort into looking their best. They are all seeking that illusive "thing" that make them happy when they look in the mirror. Despite the physical differences of the women I have seen in my aesthetics practice, the common trait is that they are all seeking what I have termed that "healthy, sexy glow." They not only want to look like themselves, they want to look like their best selves.

Women aren't wanting drastic changes; they just want to look like their premenopausal selves. That means they want to look healthy, plump, juicy, vibrant, and vital. It sounds like a lofty goal, but with advancements in products and technology, that healthy, sexy glow is much more attainable than people realize.

For many women, liking what they see in the mirror gives them a confidence boost. That confidence makes them more inclined to exercise, apply for a promotion, take a chance on a new relationship. For example, I had been telling a longtime friend and patient for years that her ice cream intake and diet of inflammatory foods was affecting her skin. I told her that if she would make those changes, she would see some positive effects. She ignored me for years. We did a chemical peel and some dermaplaning treatments on her. She saw how nice her skin could look. The next thing I knew, she was eating better and exercising. She finally saw the potential of her beauty, and she was inspired to make it a reality. This is a common theme for many of my patients. I started offering procedures, and then I realized that aesthetics increased confidence and made people happy. That happiness transcended their faces, and extended into their worlds.

MYTH

Aesthetics is limited to superficial changes
of the face and affects little else.

REALITY

As I have learned from the patients in my aesthetics chair, changing the face, even minimally, can
have exponential benefits to a woman's overall
psychological health. Time after time I have seen
women start to care for their bodies in new, more
engaged ways after aesthetics procedures.

THE TRIANGLE OF BEAUTY

Research has shown that being beautiful potentially increases salaries, improves perceptions of competency, and influences self-esteem. Even babies are partial to beautiful, symmetrical faces.[19] No wonder we all want to be beautiful! The bad news is that aging, like menopause, happens whether we're ready for it or not. The good news is that there are definitely ways to combat the physical changes using aesthetic technology. There are many procedures available that allow you to get amazing results without a facelift.

Let's talk about some of the obvious changes we go through, especially after age forty. As we age, the two things we lose in the skin are collagen and elasticity. As they decrease, the skin becomes thinner, less elastic, and ultimately wrinkled. The most precipitous drop in

---

19   Gillian Rhodes, "The Evolutionary Psychology of Facial Beauty," *Annual Rev. of Psychol.* 57, no. 1 (2006): 199–226. DOI: 10.1146/annurev. psych.57.102904.190208

collagen is between the ages of twenty-five and thirty. After thirty, we start seeing worsening sun damage, jowls, and crepey skin. These traditional signs of aging are what bring a lot of women into doctors' offices seeking treatments to turn back the hands of time.

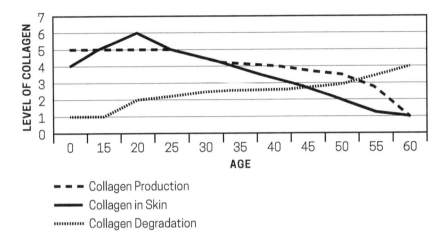

In understanding aesthetic treatments, we must understand how the face ages. A common way to describe this is the Triangle of Beauty. In a younger face, the base of the triangle is up. Our volume is in the top of our faces. As we age, we lose volume in our upper face, our temples. The fat pads shrink and migrate toward the lower face. We start to see more volume in our lower face, like jowls, hollowing of the eyes, and lines around the mouth. Blame it on collagen; blame it on gravity. That same gravity affects the face, the breasts, even the vagina.

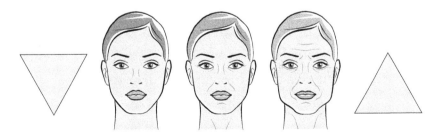

To counteract this loss of volume, there are countless noninvasive, nonsurgical treatments. Nothing is going to take the place of cutting skin and pulling it back, but if you can put enough volume and can tighten the skin, you can get similar results to a facelift. It's important to remember that even facelifts aren't permanent and they don't add volume to your face; you have to be careful about what you decide to tighten because that doesn't necessarily correct the fact that you're going to have that elasticity of skin and still need volume in certain areas, especially in your upper face to keep a natural look.

Aging is a response to inflammation, which is a culprit we have discussed throughout the book. Good diet and lifestyle habits help slow down the aging process. Smoking and an inflammatory lifestyle, on the other hand, significantly contribute to aging. This is why simply doing the Food Elimination Diet can lead to some powerful aesthetic benefits. If you're interested in exploring the different opportunities to slow the aging process, please pick your provider carefully. Look at before-and-after photos and make sure that you express your concerns before you proceed with any treatment. Also, ask for treatments that can build collagen, as opposed to just paralyzing muscles or filling the face with exogenous substances.

Skin

Before we discuss treatments that can help build volume and elasticity in your face, let's first mention one of the cheapest and most effective ways to care for your skin: sunscreen. Most of us, in our younger years, and depending on our skin shade, were not interested in protecting our skin from the sun. Sun damage is huge aging factor and can be minimized by some of the inexpensive, at-home treatments listed next.

SKIN SELF-CARE PRODUCTS

- Vitamin C—protects from free radical and sun damage

- Retinol—increases cell turnover

- Sunscreen—protects from sun damage

I encourage you to look in the mirror at the left side of your face. Now compare it to the right side of your face. For most of us who drive, the sun hits the left side of our faces more. Because of this, most people have less volume on the left side. They often have more sun spots there and more-pronounced wrinkles. Therefore, the number-one thing you should invest in is some sunscreen and a wide-brimmed hat. When you apply your sunscreen, remember that your décolletage and your hands really tell your age, so don't forget the sunscreen on these areas. Also, consider placing a sun shield on your car window and drive wearing gloves.

Aesthetics Procedures

I have the opportunity to offer patients a wide variety of aesthetics services, and for the majority of women the first procedure then motivates them to start exercising, eating well, and practicing self-care. I wouldn't believe it if I hadn't lived it. Because of my own experience with my eyebrows, I was able to have more empathy for people who had their own aesthetics issues. If it bothers you, it bothers you. And if you want to correct it, correct it. But don't feel like it's a crime to take that time or the resources because taking care of your skin is a wonderful investment. As we've mentioned above, there are things you can do at home, but there are definitely some things that you are going to want a professional to do. Let's take a closer look at some of the aesthetics options available to rejuvenate your skin.

Aesthetics Procedures:

- Dermaplaning and microdermabrasion physically exfoliate dead skin

- Chemical peels chemically exfoliate skin

- Microneedling with platelet-rich plasma (PRP) infusion (also known as the Vampire Facial)

- Fillers to replace depleted volume

- Neurotoxins (Botox™, Dysport) to decrease lines of expression

- Bio-stimulants (Sculptra and threading) to stimulate collagen beneath the skin

- Laser/skin resurfacing: Damages skin to stimulate rejuvenated skin and increase collagen production and elasticity

One of the most well-known aesthetics treatments is Botox injections. Neurotoxins in the end are "Band-Aids" to cover up the reality that your skin has lost collagen and elasticity. On the other hand, however, I love to see patients presenting for neurotoxins, because it's a wonderful opportunity to address what's REALLY happening to their skin. Neurotoxins are wonderful "entry drugs" into the world of aesthetics. You can try Botox all you want, but at some point, it's just a matter of volume; this is why the aesthetic industry is going through a change and creating therapies that aim to create collagen. The industry is recognizing that by helping people build and maintain their own collagen, they achieve a more natural look.

MYTH

Adding Botox or fillers will make me look unnatural.

REALITY

The aesthetics industry has made huge advancements in therapies available to women who want to look natural. The aesthetics of today, when done correctly, leave you looking like yourself. Only better. The reason people look unnatural is not specific to the products but rather to products used and the technique of the injector.

One option to build and maintain collagen is collagen induction injection treatments like microneedling. With this treatment, we can use different substances, like hyaluronic acid or platelet-rich plasma (PRP). With PRP, we draw your blood and centrifuge it down. Then we take the platelet-rich portion part of it, which has growth factors, and either infuse it back into the skin through the micro channels that are created through the microneedling, or we actually inject it into areas where we want to see more collagen growth and elasticity. Think of the microneedling as aerating the soil and the PRP as fertilizer.

Another treatment option is injecting fillers, such as hyaluronic acid or calcium hydroxyapatite. We can also inject collagen-inducing substances such as L-polylactic acid (like Sculptra Aesthetic). This is actually one of my favorite treatments, because it doesn't just fill up areas that have lost volume, but it strategically places collagen-inducing agents in key places, per the Triangle of Beauty.

Another popular treatment is threading, in which we introduce threads under the skin. The threads are similar to fabric, and basically they cause an inflammatory reaction under the skin. This inflammatory reaction causes the skin to induce/create more collagen fibers.

There are also superficial ways to treat with laser treatments. One of the best anti-aging treatments that women can start doing is intense pulsed light (IPL). This is technically not a laser, but it is a light treatment. It micro-damages the skin through heat. Patients who have done this type of light therapy often have better skin than when they were young because it reduces fine lines and builds collagen and elasticity on the surface of the skin. This treatment is only available for women with lighter complexions. The darker you are, the more careful you need to be with laser therapies. However, there are several more advanced lasers on the market to treat women of color.

Heat therapies are very successful in inducing collagen and tightening skin. When performed appropriately in patients that do not have severe laxity, microfocused ultrasound heat (Ultherapy TM) can yield results similar to a facelift. The downside is that the results are short-lived, two to three years maximum. Remember, though, with any type of collagen-induction therapy, it takes weeks to months to see a difference because it's not an immediate fix. You are literally changing the protein nature of the tissue. As you can imagine, that takes a while to manifest outwardly in the skin. A similar heat therapy is using a radio frequency heat treatment called ThermiTight and Thermage. With this therapy, we can stay superficially on the skin or take a probe and go directly under the skin, which can tighten up skin and burn fat.

The Fat Tire

Although aesthetic services are often associated with the face, some therapies address other common complaints in menopausal women. You knew we'd address it eventually: the dreaded "fat tire." The bad news is that it happens, the good news is that it happens to women and men. That seems fair, right? As we age, we gain fat, and the fat deposits in certain areas, especially the lower abdomen. I can't count the number of women who come in my office, grab their tires, and exclaim "What is this? Where did it come from?"

The most obvious treatment is through a healthy diet and exercise. But I will be honest, it's some stubborn fat. As we age, we have to do more to maintain our weight. You read that right—just to maintain. What you used to be able to do to lose weight is now what you have to do just to keep what you have. And I think that's one of the hardest realities to face, that your caloric requirements are lower, your energy requirements are higher, and your metabolism declines in part because of your thyroid.

Your physical activity becomes more important as you age, and it's never too late to start moving and eating better. There's no getting around it. Alcohol and the foods that we tend to gravitate toward when we're stressed and depressed are the exact things that feed that fat tire.

There are, however, some effective treatments that can minimize or diminish a fat tire. One of my favorite treatments to get rid of this stubborn fat is CoolSculpting. It freezes the fat, and then the fat dies through a process called *apoptosis*, which is permanent. Once you kill a cell, it's not coming back. I have seen some profound changes in patients who have opted for CoolScuplting.

In the event that you want to address the stubborn fat, there are several noninvasive modalities that target fat cells and can permanently remove them. These treatments, though not for everyone, help minimize the lower abdominal fat that is such a common complaint among aging women and men.

***

I had a friend in high school who would always say, "Black don't crack." I never understood what she meant until I started to age and see the difference between me and my counterparts with less-melanated skin. But despite having some great genes and the advantage of darker skin, I have seen dramatic results with my skin by following the simple steps of exfoliating (chemical peels) and inducing collagen (microneedling). Furthermore, by removing toxic relationships and stressful work environments in combination with healthy diet and skin care basics, I have seen a drastic improvement in my skin. Most people don't think that I have had anything done to my skin. But I always respond, "Are you kidding? I've done it *all* to my face." The whole point is doing it subtly, and doing it in a way that keeps you in a good place, and not taking it over the top. Nobody wants to look like they've had something done; everybody merely wants to keep what they have.

Look, you're going to age. It's your decision how you want to care for yourself in your later years. In the end, what you look like matters, probably mostly to you. Countless women in my chair have proclaimed that they are going to just give up the fight and let the wrinkle boogeyman claim it all. They are torn by the expense of trying to maintain or at least keep the wrinkles at bay, and knowing that in the end they will be judged by their appearance in the workplace, among their peers, and even, and more unfortunately, in their relationships. I am often conflicted by providing a service that both benefits my patient's self-esteem and concurrently adds to a systemic problem. That said, there is nothing more gratifying than witnessing a woman's beautiful transformation from an aging face to one that appears ten years younger.

Taking care of your looks doesn't mean that you neglect your spiritual or your personal growth. On the contrary. Taking care of your physical self can be the match that lights the fire to get you back to your personal best, whatever that is for you. It's harder to be your personal best if you don't like what you see in the mirror. You either have to change the perception or change what you see. The decision to entertain aesthetic procedures should be for you and not to meet a beauty standard set by your partner or culture. It should come from a place of wanting to live your most authentic life and love what you see in your reflection. Take care of your body and your outer beauty. It's not vanity. It's accepting and even enjoying the process of aging and continuing to be the vibrant person you've always been.

> **Taking care of your physical self can be the match that lights the fire to get you back to your personal best, whatever that is for you.**

CLOSING TAKEAWAYS

1. If you're interested in exploring aesthetic services, pick your provider carefully. Look at before-and-after photos and make sure you express your concerns before you proceed with any treatment.

2. One of the cheapest and most effective ways to care for your skin is by using sunscreen daily on your face, chest, and backs of hands.

3. Don't feel like it's a crime to spend time and resources on your looks, because taking care of your skin is a wonderful investment.

4. The aesthetics industry is recognizing that by helping people build and maintain their own collagen, they achieve a more natural look.

5. It's not the products that are used that make people look unnatural. Injector technique is the number-one indicator of how well an aesthetics treatment will look.

CHAPTER 8

REBIRTH AND REINVENTION: JEWELS FOR THE JOURNEY

What I have learned on my own menopausal journey is that self-mastery is one of the most important tools needed to achieve rebirth and reinvention. Like myself, you can be quite knowledgeable about what you *should* do, but that's not the same as doing it. Self-mastery is the ability to apply what we know into what we actually do. So, I know a lot of things:

- I KNOW that eating wheat and dairy leads to me feeling sluggish, having joint pain, and experiencing irregular digestion.

- I KNOW that thirty to forty-five minutes of cardio exercise makes me feel better and helps me keep my weight down and my mood up!

- I KNOW that it takes longer to arrive at destinations than I routinely plan.

- I KNOW that honoring a daily morning spiritual practice brings an unparalleled sense of peace and centeredness.

> Self-mastery is the ability to discipline our thoughts and actions and routinely align what we KNOW with how we ACT.

But how does what we know translate into daily routines and habits? Self-mastery is the ability to discipline our thoughts and actions and routinely align what we KNOW with how we ACT. Like many of us, I continue to juggle responsibilities: family, patients, my business. What's missing from this list? Ah, yes: me. Self-care is like flossing your teeth—you know you need to do it, it doesn't take long, and *not doing it* can cause further health issues. Like flossing, you don't necessarily see the consequences until you go to a doctor and hear the dreaded news that you have compromised health or a disease. By that point, it can be too late.

In preparing to write this chapter, I realized this might be the hardest piece to practice—self-care. As I looked critically at my own life, I realized I wasn't walking the walk. I'm not getting things done, because I'm just going, going, going. I never want to take a day off because I don't want to lose the revenue or disappoint my patients. Despite any nobility of my reasons, my body doesn't care. It needs a break.

I have carved out days in my schedule to devote to my self-care. I go to the gym, the dentist, get my mammogram, whatever it is that's just for me that day. I don't allow myself an excuse, because, believe me, there is always an excuse. I instinctively know what I need to do, but like the rest of us, I'm still trying to figure out how to do it. At the end of the day self-care requires one thing and one thing only, *discipline*.

SELF-CARE AND BALANCE

An inflammatory lifestyle includes not only the food that we eat, but also the activities that we engage in and the thoughts that we think. Meditation, exercise, and participating in joyful activities are all anti-inflammatory. They're all stress reducing, and anything that reduces stress is going to reduce inflammation. We've already discussed the physical ramifications of stress and how it increases your severity and susceptibility to disease, decreases your immune responsiveness, and diminishes wound healing. From a medical standpoint, the whole point of self-care is to help manage stress so you can be alive. But there are also bigger, more spiritual and personal reasons to take care of yourself.

MYTH

Self-care is not mandatory to my health and well-being.

REALITY

Self-care is one of the best, most proactive things you can do for your own health. It has systemic benefits on your body, your mood, your energy levels, and beyond.

My practice is named Tula Wellness, because *tula* means "balance" in Sanskrit. It is so important to consider the imbalances in our lives. I try to educate my patients about the ways their daily stressors and relationships can affect their health. Small things can alter the balance in our lives—traffic, stressful jobs, obsessive thoughts, troubled relationships. These are all inflammatory situations, and as we learned in chapter 6, these can lead to disease and chronic conditions. These events, both big and small, create a physiological response in us. Our bodies were meant to react to foreign bodies and stress for short periods of time; we're not designed, however, for this prolonged inflammatory response. Our culture is so attached to social media and work and other obligations that we've created an environment rife with inflammatory triggers that leave little time or space for repair and restoration. This is why we are seeing higher instances of cancer, depression, and neurological diseases.

Real Talk

Let's be real: women usually put themselves at the bottom of their to-do list, which is why self-care *seems* like such a radical concept, when, in fact, it should be the norm. Some of this is circumstantial—we have work and families and laundry and cooking and bills and budgeting and errands. Some of it, however, is a choice.

I know this is an unpopular message, but women need to take ownership for our own martyrdom. Why do we carry our exhaustion around like badges of honor? Why does it feel good, even unconsciously, to be needed by so many people? I've had conversations with countless women who tell me they just don't have time. They have too many people depending on them.

Women need to be more aware and critical of the cultural messages we receive. You can't watch fifteen minutes of television without seeing commercials that glorify "super women." We see images of women at the helm of board meetings, then at home lovingly removing laundry stains and wiping runny noses. Where are the messages empowering women to draw a bath, lock the door, and tell her family to stand back for ten minutes? Cultural messages tell us that we should be strong, capable in all areas, and have an inexhaustible supply of energy for others. This is a dangerous message that seeps into our collective psyche and creates false expectations that we *should* be able to manage it all.

Conversely, there is another cultural message, much older than the super-woman archetype of recent history, that is just as damaging and misleading—the damsel. From childhood, we are told stories of women being rescued by someone. We all know the tale. The woman is in peril, or in a deep slumber, when a handsome prince shows up and literally sweeps her off her feet to carry her back to his castle where he will take care of her. Most women might recoil from the thought of being a kept woman, but for many of us, the thought of someone else taking over is magnificent. Why? Because we try to be super women! We try to do it all. Maybe the fantasy is less about the romance and more about the dissolution of the responsibilities we (willingly) take on.

MYTH

One day, the perfect partner will rescue me and make life complete.

REALITY

Not. Gonna. Happen. It's time to rescue yourself.

These messages aren't even close to the reality. The reality is that in at least 40 percent of households in the United States women are the primary breadwinners.[20] I will admit, there are days when the thought of a handsome, tall, thoughtful, sensitive, caring, rich man who wants to take care of me sounds pretty nice. If he showed up, I

---

20 Sarah Jane Glynn, "Breadwinning Mothers Are Increasingly the U.S. Norm," Center for American Progress, accessed May 1, 2019, https://www. americanprogress.org/issues/women/reports/2016/12/19/295203/ breadwinning-mothers-are-increasingly-the-u-s-norm/.

might swoon with the best of the princesses. But, I'm a realist, and I want to empower women to be emotionally self-sufficient, because the "Rescuer" is just a fantasy. If you're waiting for the prince, good luck with that. You need to take care of yourself. That's not a message we're often told, and if it is, it's not a message easily heard.

We must find the balance between being the damsel princess waiting for rescue and the superhero woman rescuing everyone else. Finding the balance within that spectrum is difficult and changes daily. This all might sound harsh, but I want to remind women that it doesn't have to be this way. I'm not here to debate our culture. We are products of our time. Cultural evolution is a glacial process. It happens painfully slow over generations. But there is hope. Rather than being reactive to the stereotypes, let's be proactive.

> ## Let's take ownership of our own complicated relationship with martyrdom.

Let's take ownership of our own complicated relationship with martyrdom. Let's accept that it feels good to be needed and wanted by our families. Let's also accept that you can't be selfless all the time without resentment. This is not a topic women like to discuss, but, yes, you resent your children. Of course you love them and choose to accommodate their needs, but you're fooling yourself if you don't think that it doesn't come with a price. The more you give, the more resentment you may feel because you're closing off your own dreams, your own hopes, your own brilliance.

Even as I write this book, I struggle with this. I've had the dream inside of me for a long time to write this book, but writing it takes me away from my family. It takes my focus, my energy, my time. Should I be solely focused on my children? After all, there is an unspoken sentiment that how our children turn out has everything to do with the time and guidance they received. We do our best so we can raise spectacular children and get a gold star upon completion. Nothing like a serving of mommy guilt when taking time to feed your soul.

It is natural and normal to resent the trappings of your life. Family life can be a beautiful cage. We are creatures that have the mental capacity to hold opposing truths. In fact, some psychologists claim that that's the definition of psychological health. When you associate yourself with martyrdom, but deny the resentment that can often accompany it, then you are stuffing some emotions deep down. Furthermore, when you give yourself little to no time to check in with yourself to identify and work through these emotions, they can resurface physically through illness and disease. In fact, if your cup is empty, you can't fill anyone else's cup. It always reminds me of the airplane safety warnings to put your own oxygen mask on first before assisting others. The hard truth is you're not a super woman. And, besides, that little cape comes with a large price.

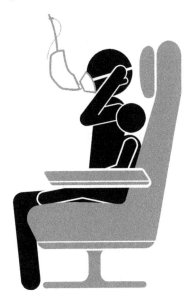

When it comes to self-care, it's on you. Spoiler alert: no one is coming to rescue you. I don't want to sound harsh, but I do want to encourage a generation of empowered and woke women who can rescue themselves through self-care. As we age, we continue to be the primary providers of care. We add partners, children, pets, aging parents. But who's taking care of you? Nobody's taking care of you. Your husband's not taking care of you. Your kids aren't taking care of you. Your mother's not taking care of you. Your friends aren't taking care of you. This isn't to say that you don't rely on these important people and benefit greatly from the support and encouragement, but there is a real expectation that *you* will take care of *them*.

I believe that people respect you more when you have clear boundaries. Nobody respects someone they can walk all over. You allow other people to come into your space. You're the one who has to set the boundary, and if you haven't set them for twenty years, then you can't be mad that people don't respect the threshold now. You have to gently reestablish the boundary until all the people who depend on you accept it and respect it. You can't do it by slamming the door when you're pissed off, without explaining the limits to people. Calmly state that you need fifteen minutes alone. When family members forget or they screw up (which they will), gently remind them until they get it right. If you revere the routine, then they'll revere the routine. You can't expect others to honor you when you don't honor yourself. Once again, this is why I named my practice Tula Wellness, because we are all, me included, constantly striving toward a balanced life.

Radical Self-Care

The radical aspect of self-care is that it is unapologetic. I know that's not something that is traditionally encouraged in women, and I'm not saying it will come easily at first, but you must claim some time for yourself. Snatch it up and don't share it with anyone. It doesn't mean you don't love the people around you, it just means you love yourself as well.

When my kids were younger, I made an actual sign that I would hang on my door when I needed some time to myself. I didn't do anything fancy with this time usually. I just wanted to sit in a room in silence. My family learned that when my sign was on the door, much like a "Do Not Disturb" sign in a hotel, I was unavailable. Mommy was on break. I encourage you to make a literal or figurative sign that alerts those around you that you are taking a break, and you're not apologizing for it. Again, taking some time to yourself is not radical; doing it without regret is.

RULES OF SELF-CARE
- No Shame
- No Apologies
- No Guilt
- No Explanations
- No Excuses

RITUAL, ROUTINE, READY SET GO!

A balanced lifestyle must involve mindfulness and a slowed pace. But it's not just doing it once a month or once a year. In order to reap the benefits of self-care, you must make it sacred through ritual and routine. If we can incorporate more intentional habits in our lives, then they become routines, thus creating a mentally and physically healthy lifestyle.

One of my daily rituals is the simple act of taking a bath. When I'm in the bathtub, even if it's just five minutes in the morning, I lock the door, I'm quiet, I play soft music. This is a sacred time for me and

I use it for prayer, grounding, and stress management. It's also an important way to make time for myself. That's *my* time. I feel like something's missing if I don't sit in the tub, because that is my little safe space. My husband will want to come in, and I answer, "Nope. This is my five minutes. I'm sorry. Nobody can come in, not even you." After my bath, I usually anoint myself with essential oils. I place oils on different body points, whether it's my wrist or behind my ear or at the crown of my head, to serve as reminders to stay grounded and to set intentions for the day.

> **Sometimes, changing the health of your body starts with changing the health of your mind.**

Rituals are an integral part of self-care and mindfulness. Sometimes, changing the health of your body starts with changing the health of your mind. It's a great practice to create small rituals for yourself that remind you to be mindful and still. Sometimes, we wake up, start moving, and we never stop until bedtime. Without rituals, and intentional mindfulness, it can feel like life throws us around. If rituals are not built into our daily processes, it's easy to skip them. Think small. An important ritual can be as easy as kneeling by the bed and thinking of one thing you're grateful for.

You can create a ritual around anything that you do—tea, bath, yoga, running, vacuuming, walking. Remind yourself to be mindful, quiet, and reflective. Don't think of your to-do list, your grocery list, your responsibilities. Empty your mind and be present to what is happening now.

In *The Artist's Way,* Julia Cameron discusses the powerful transformation that can come from creating a daily ritual around what she calls "Morning Pages." She advises readers to wake each morning and write several pages. It doesn't matter what you write. It doesn't matter if it's any good. It doesn't matter if you or anyone else ever reads it. This simple act of journaling each day can transform the way you think and ease the stress and inflammation in your body. It also has the added benefit of helping you to get in touch with yourself, your joys, your fears. There isn't a magic formula for self-care. Some people might like something active like running, others might prefer quiet tai chi or massage.

Whatever you choose, stick with it. Don't bail. You would never miss your kid's doctor appointments; you would never cancel a meeting with your boss. Give your self-care the same reverence and priority.

HOW DOES SELF-CARE LOOK TO YOU?

- Energy medicine
- Yoga
- Gardening
- Hot baths
- Dancing
- Therapy
- Tai Chi
- Prayer
- Meditation
- Acupuncture
- Journaling
- Walking

I find that when I am doing certain procedures on patients, such as injecting fillers, I'm literally able to meditate. I put music on, focus on facial artistry, and get in the zone. Injecting filler and restoring somebody's face—combining science and art—is like painting a picture. Even though it's work, it brings me joy. For me, a lot of my joy is connected to my work, and that's okay. If your work brings you joy, it's validation that you are living your passion. You're living what you want to see for your life. If going to work brings you joy, then that's what brings you joy. No judgment. Even in work, you can find ways to let go of the trappings of daily life and just *be*.

MYTH

What does self-care have to do with my health?

REALITY

It *is* your health.

Establishing methods of self-care is really about finding your joy. One of the things we ask in our Tula Wellness patient intake questionnaire is what brings a person joy. Some new patients balk at the question and are surprised when they don't have an answer. "What does this have to do with my health?" My answer is simply, "It *is* your health." If you can't answer that question, then you need to give yourself time and space to find the answer. Is it painting? Is it swimming? Is it driving long distances? Is it playing with your dog? Whatever it is, you need to identify it so you can make sure that you incorporate it into your daily self-care routine.

Finding Your Joy

What brings you joy?

God, Jesus, My husband, Children, family, hair, make up Clothes, My job & Exercise. Time to fit healthy!!

How often do you engage in this activity?

Every day!

How might you change your schedule or priorities to do this activity more often? Don't need a to, I already am doing it.

Write out your activity in a ritualistic way. Describe each step of the activity. GOD & JESUS

FOCUS We got this!!

151

Often, people tell me they watch television or use electronics for self-care. I'm not here to judge, and I've certainly been known to spend some time on Words with Friends or binge on Netflix, but electronics typically inhibit the practice of going inward and being reflective. Don't mistake self-care with zoning out from the world, because there's a difference between being in a meditative, joyful state versus checking out from reality and disassociating from yourself. Self-medicating with alcohol and drugs or even video games and TV do nothing for allowing us to truly go inward and hear our quiet voices. When it comes to restoring yourself, make sure you're checking in, not out. Sometimes, you don't feel like finding your joy. Sometimes, you just need to check out, and that's okay too.

> **Don't mistake self-care with zoning out from the world.**

JEWELS FOR THE JOURNEY

Self-care is taking a moment to stop and do something for ourselves. We've talked about the importance of ritual and routine, but self-care also includes the hard work of self-discipline. Sometimes, it's hard to check in for self-care. Sometimes, it's like *I don't even know what I need to do for myself because I'm just so tired. I don't even have anything to even give myself.* To help me establish this self-care discipline, even in times of exhaustion, I created a self-care guide called Jewels for the Journey. The jewels help you to get into this space of joy and being. It gives you a road map to help you practice having discipline and boundaries.

JEWELS FOR THE JOURNEY

- Gratitude ✓
- Acceptance ✓
- Purity ✓
- Self-care ✓
- Prayer ✓
- Silence ✓
- Vision ✓
- Service ✓
- Love ✓
- Discipline ✓

Gratitude

The discipline of self-care starts with gratitude. We can get caught up in the political strife and violence of our culture, and at some point, we have to stop and acknowledge that amid this conflict and vitriol, there is much to be grateful for. When we forget gratitude, the world becomes something to fear and battle against. You must focus on what is good to create a calm worldview for yourself and your family.

Acceptance

Why is it so hard to accept things as they are? This is such an important step in the self-care process and allows you let go of stress and mental noise about things you have little to no control over. For me, I accept the fact that I have teenagers right now, and with that comes a certain amount of delinquency and irritation. I don't like it, but I just accept that this is the phase I'm in, and I don't need to fight it because I will never win. Accept what is; accept what is not. This might require you to read some books or seek therapy. Sometimes, this involves some grieving. Allow yourself to experience the feelings and then you're free to release the emotions and fill that new open space with joy and acceptance.

Purity

Purity is about keeping your mind, thoughts, relationships, and body pure. If you're going to continually watch violent television, or think negative thoughts, it's going to alter your worldview and inform your decision-making. You can achieve this purity of thought through scriptures, self-help books, meditation, or anything else that infuses you with positivity. Don't forget that purity of body is also important. When you're stressed, you might reach for a cookie, which is the opposite comfort you need. Keep your diet clean and reach for wholesome foods when you're stressed. But, and this is important, sometimes you just need to eat the damn cookie! If that's the case, accept that you ate it and then move along. There is no room for self-flagellation in the self-care protocol.

Prayer

For me, prayer is a general term that requires asking. It doesn't matter *who* you're asking—God, the Universe, a Higher Power, Allah, Buddha, whoever or whatever you believe in. The important part of this step is the asking. It's a shift in perspective to humble yourself before a source that is greater than you and asking for peace, guidance, and help. The simple step of asking can create powerful shifts in perception that can put the daily stressors of life into a refreshingly cosmic-sized perspective.

Silence

If prayer is about asking, silence is about listening. Silence means putting yourself in a state of attentive listening. You can listen to your Higher Spirit, Inner Child, God, whatever it is that's talking to you.

You have to be still enough to listen; if you're not going do that, then you can't hear. There's so much that you could have if you just stop, ask, and listen. I know it sounds really simple. And it is. Try it, and you'll be amazed.

Vision

We don't know where we're headed if we're not looking ahead. We need to create a vision for what we want to see in our lives. For this reason, I'm a fan of vision boards. These simple boards can be powerful tools for bringing your abstract hopes and dreams into concrete realities. How many of us really sit down and ask ourselves, *What do I want?* You can't *have* what you want when you don't *know* what you want. For every vision board I've ever made, I've gotten what I want. For example, I once made a vision board early in my practice. I had no money because I was building Tula Wellness. When I was making my vision board, I added Italy. I knew there was no way financially I could make it happen, but I added it anyway because I *wanted* it to happen. I *asked* for it to happen. Within six months of that vision board, I was in Italy. I don't even know exactly how it happened, but when it did, I accepted it and was grateful for it. I can't tell you how important creating a vision is to seeing the change show up in your life.

Service

As anyone who has ever been in a rut knows, it's a self-centered mind-set. When you get in this cycle, you might think, *My job is bad, my family is fractured, my life is off course.* As you see here, the theme is *my, my, my.* The unwelcome but often-sobering antidote to that woeful selfishness is asking yourself, *What am I doing for others?* I don't mean your normal nurturing, mothering role, I mean for a bigger cause—your community, your city, your world. If we can go to that place of servitude, it shifts us from being self-centered to service-centered. We get so accustomed to our daily inconveniences that we sometimes think they actually are meaningful. When my kids start complaining of dirty Converse sneakers or my second car needs a tune-up, I can get lost in these annoyances, or I can go and witness real inconvenience at a shelter or soup kitchen. Much like prayer, service is helpful because it shifts your focus. It's not about you, it's about others. It feels counterintuitive when you're in the dark cycle of self-loathing, but an attitude and practice of servitude can be a profound antidote to a depressive state.

Love

This aspect of self-care speaks for itself, though not in the way I want to highlight it here: self-love. This is one concept that might seem radical when put into practice, but again, it shouldn't be radical. It should be natural, normal, and welcomed by those around you. Part of showing yourself self-love is surrounding yourself with people who support you and bring you peace and happiness. As I've mentioned already, midlife is often a time when women look closely at their relationships. You will have friends who don't take care of themselves. Often, these are the friends who make you feel guilty when you have rigid boundaries around your self-care. I like to think it's not malicious; it's a call for help. Either way, surround yourself with friends who respect your self-love. The same goes for romantic partners. Your partner must at least accept and respect your self-care routines, whether they agree with it or not. Self-love can be what swoops in and saves your inner damsel. Be your own hero.

Discipline

You're going to slip up, you're going to forget, you're going to get into another rut, you're going to be tired, and you're going to find reasons not to enact these self-care strategies. This is where discipline is a useful tool. Discipline is the reminder that when you get to the bottom of the list, you go right back up to Gratitude and do it all over again. Discipline reminds you to ask yourself *How can I honor myself today?* Make sure you follow through with yourself, just as you would for a friend or child you'd made promises to.

BE JUICY!

Luckily some of the tools mentioned in this chapter become an inner drive, whether we're aware of them or not. As our hormones and biochemistry change in midlife, so too do our priorities and expectations. Your body and soul are hungry to execute these self-care strategies. The following steps to self-care will continue to serve you on your path to balance.

STEPS TO SELF-CARE
- Ownership
- Boundaries
- Authenticity
- Eating to live

As we enter into this second half of life, we have all these aforementioned tools to work with, but we sometimes continue to procrastinate. We continue to need permission. I think this is why women are twice as likely to develop an autoimmune disease.[21] Often, the

---

21   DeLisa Fairweather and Noel R. Rose, "Women and Autoimmune Diseases," *Emerging Infectious Diseases* 10, no. 11 (Nov. 2004), 2005–2011.

only way we get to escape is if we're sick or dead. It benefits us to be sick in this way. It's a boundary; it is permission. Regardless of the circumstances, you have to do the work. There's no formula out there for you. There's no instant solution. There's no easy pill. If you're not willing to do the work, then just accept that and know there will be certain health and lifestyle challenges that you'll have as a result. I feel like some of the angst and irritation women feel during this time is because they're not living their truth. They're not living their vital, juicy, authentic lives. They're just emotionally dead because they've not nurtured themselves.

Often, I have older women who come into my office with tales of empty nests and deceased partners, and they will have an epiphany one day and proclaim to me, "I'm ready. I'm ready to live." Just recently a seventy-year-old patient came into my office. She had been taking care of her husband for more than a decade before he died. She came in unburdened by caretaking. She told me she had started caring for *herself.* She said, "Wow. There's still something there, there's still a lot left!" She was surprised to find herself rejuvenated by this new care she was honoring herself with. It was almost as if this woman was falling in love with herself. She was being her own hero and saving herself. It was beautiful to behold.

As I've mentioned, one of the most beautiful aspects of menopause is letting go of the shame and fear of what other people might think. There are some people who, even before age fifty, didn't really care what people thought. I wasn't one of those people, but as I'm getting older, it is so liberating to let that go. We can take our hormones, go to the doctor, check our thyroids, but we are not well and balanced until we fix our thoughts and make a decision—how are we going to embrace the juicy second half of our lives? There is no getting around the work that needs to be done. The work of healing is the work of tapping into self and being honest with the changes that need to be made. If we don't make the intentional, conscious effort to create a different reality, then it's not going to change.

While counseling women, I'm struck by some's unwillingness to accept the fact that, as we age, we must change. Change can be scary and difficult, but it's the path to personal growth and evolution. You can't get your healing until you do your work. Despite how you care for yourself and the ways you choose to practice that, all that matters is that you're living your truth, and doing what's good for you and your family. It is time to own your brilliance and claim your juicy life. Taste the flavor, extract the juice, get all the joy you can from living and being.

CLOSING TAKEAWAYS

1. Daily events, both big and small, create a physiological response in us. Our bodies were meant to react to foreign bodies and stress for short periods of time; we're not designed, however, for this prolonged inflammatory response.

2. Self-care is a choice. Claim some time for yourself. Snatch it up and don't share it with anyone.

3. Be mindful and cautious of cultural messages that tell you to be strong, capable in all areas, and have an inexhaustible supply of energy for others. This is a dangerous message that sets you up for failure.

4. Take ownership of your own complicated relationship with martyrdom.

5. When you give yourself little to no time to check in with yourself to identify and work through dark emotions, they can resurface physically through illness and disease.

6. People respect you more when you have clear boundaries.

7. In order to reap the benefits of self-care, you must make it sacred through ritual and routine.

THE MENOPAUSE REVOLUTION

Midlife is when the universe gently places her hands upon your shoulders, pulls you close, and whispers in your ear:

I'm not screwing around. All of this pretending and performing—these coping mechanisms that you've developed to protect yourself from feeling inadequate and getting hurt—has to go. Your armor is preventing you from growing into your gifts. I understand that you needed these protections when you were small. I understand that you believed your armor could help you secure all of the things you needed to feel worthy and lovable, but you're still searching and you're more lost than ever. Time is growing short. There are unexplored adventures ahead of you. You can't live the rest of your life worried about what other people think. You were born worthy of love and belonging.

Courage and daring are coursing through your veins. You were made to live and love with your whole heart. It's time to show up and be seen.[22] —Brené Brown

There's something that starts brewing in our forties and fifties—the uneasy reality that if we are not living our dreams by now, there are fewer vibrant years before us than behind us. I certainly felt this with regard to writing this book. I have been ruminating on this book for the past twenty-five years. I thought a lot about my journey that began at midlife and what it has meant for my personal evolution. I questioned how much of an "unraveling," as author Brené Brown calls it, I have already gone through, and how much I have left. I even questioned if I was worthy enough to speak on such an immense topic. Full disclosure: I'm teaching what I still have to learn. I am myself in the middle of the confusion, angst, reinvention, brilliance, and blossoming pulled along by the deep knowing that more of my life has passed than is in front of me; but there is still so much to do. What could I possibly have to offer in the midst of so much information that is already available? Despite my insecurities, the call to write this book whispered in my ear and became too loud to ignore.

Part of the impetus for this book was my own life-changing peri/menopausal symptoms and the arduous journey toward naming them. Over the years, however, as I had countless conversations with women about the myths and realities of menopause, it became more apparent that I *had* to write this book. I knew there were women, like me, whose lives changed after age thirty-five: Did they too feel like they were going crazy? Were they having scary thoughts about their partners? Were they gaining weight and feeling miserable about themselves without knowing why? I realized I could fill in the blanks

---

22 Brené Brown, "The Midlife Unraveling," *On Midlife*, May 24, 2018, https://brenebrown.com/blog/2018/05/24/the-midlife-unraveling/.

for these women. I could inform them of all the realities of life after age thirty-five that their mothers, doctors, and friends hadn't told them. I knew that if I did not write the book *now*, I might never. I kept thinking about the noble endeavor to uplift women, and though it seems Herculean, I couldn't ignore it any longer. The universe kept nudging. So, at age fifty-one, I stopped waiting on an outside rescuer, put on my big-girl panties, and stepped into the life I always knew was waiting for me.

I realize that I am writing about one of the most critical periods of a woman's life journey. A common theme of the peri/menopausal phase is conflict. Women in dead-end relationships and jobs are some of the unhappiest women you'll meet. As we mature and our hormones fluctuate, and especially as estrogen levels decline, the veil is lifted. We see things with a new clarity and begin to assess where we are in life. By age fifty, it is apparent that if you have not started making a plan to create the life you really want for yourself, then you may never live it. There are hard realities associated with wearing your big-girl panties. There is no comfort in complicity.

The real change—the real menopause—is about growing into your own life. It's about embracing the boldness, the frailty, the passion, the grief, the joy, the suffering, and every other emotion that brought you to this place. The change is accepting the sacred knowing that we are here for passion and purpose. The pain of menopause is the resistance to coming into our own.

The pain of menopause is the resistance to coming into our own.

In dispelling the myths that have existed around menopause for generations, we are taking ownership of a transformative time in our lives. We are creating a menopause revolution. This revolution is being ushered in by *unsilenced* women. I use this term to describe the women—from millennials to baby boomers—who are no longer quiet when it comes to their bodies and the changes they experience. They are the women who will not be silenced by tradition, decorum, or previously held myths. They want the realities. They will not accept that conversations regarding their bodies and sexual pleasures are taboo. I am one of these women, and I hope to raise and inspire these women. I hope to start as many conversations as I can about women's health and the powerful transformations we go through.

The realities of women's menopausal experiences have been kept silenced for too long. Not anymore. There is an awakening happening in our culture surrounding women's experiences, and this extends to all realms, including those of health, sexuality, and maturity. This movement, led by women who seek understanding, pleasure, and vitality especially in the second half of life, is leading to a powerful awakening for all women. This knowledge about and acceptance of the realities of our natural, normal female evolution allows us to dispel the myths that have kept us disconnected from our bodies and our experiences for generations. With understanding of our bodies comes acceptance of our evolving power throughout life and is the catalyst that will change the landscape of women's health and carry forth the power of the menopause revolution. Are you ready?

WHEN WILL YOU BE READY?

When will you be ready

To see your own greatness?

To move your own mountains?

There are no more excuses

Only the possibility

to live your best life

Only the knowing of Spirit

that speaks to you

Spirit that knows

Spirit that guides

Pull up your passion.

Confront your fear.

DECIDE that you are ready

and MOVE.

–Dr. Arianna Sholes-Douglas

A WORD ABOUT VAGINAL REJUVENATION

I am happy to say that one of fastest-growing fields in medicine is female vaginal rejuvenation. With these technologies, we're trying to restore the vagina to its previous function. The main method of doing this is through building collagen.

Collagen is not just for the face anymore. Building collagen is important in both aesthetics and female intimate health. The purpose of collagen-building is to restore vaginal function. The term that has been used for this field has been *rejuvenation*, but I think that's going to change in the coming years because it doesn't speak to what's really happening, which is restoring the vagina to its previous state. Perhaps the term *vaginal restoration* is more appropriate.

VAGINAL REJUVENATION THERAPY

- CO2 laser
- Erbium YAG
- Radiofrequency
- Stem cell, platelet-rich plasma
- Pelvic floor rehabilitation
- Surgical procedures: Labiaplasty of labia minora/majora, vaginal tightening

There are multiple modalities currently being used for vaginal rejuvenation. The most common modalities are CO2 laser and radiofrequency heat. CO2 laser works by superficially affecting the outer layer of tissue. This treatment utilizes laser applicators that will literally ablate the vaginal lining, internally and externally. These treatments are growing in popularity. And although the entire experience of a woman should be considered (hormones, diet, hormone replacement therapy) any and all types of providers including dermatologist, plastic surgeons, and even aesthetics centers are jumping on the bandwagon.

Radiofrequency is another popular treatment. Like other vaginal rejuvenation techniques, radiofrequency helps to create collagen. That collagen is increasing the glycogen and the ability of the cells to turn over and create lubrication. These procedures can also dramatically improve urinary incontinence. In fact, radiofrequency and CO2 laser are tools urologists are using to treat incontinence as opposed to invasive surgical procedures. So, instead of invasive treatment, especially with women with mild to moderate incontinence, we can use radiofrequency as a treatment.

Stem cell therapy/platelet-rich plasma (PRP) is another technology used for vaginal restoration. One technology injects PRP back into the body to produce collagen (also known as O Shot™). The PRP is obtained by drawing blood, spinning it down, removing the platelet-rich portion of the plasma, and injecting it into the clitoris and/or peri-urethral/G-spot.

There's no significant evidence that combining the therapies is superior, but I have found that when we combine CO2 laser, radio-frequency, and PRP, or even stem cells, we can get enhanced results. But there is still a lot of research needed to validate these treatments and ensure that there are no long-term effects.

VAGINAL REJUVENATION

- Increases vaginal moisture
- Strengthens vaginal muscles
- Improves painful intercourse
- Reduces urinary leakages and urgency
- Improves vaginal looseness
- Increases vaginal sensitivity

After patients have received vaginal rejuvenation therapies, they often comment that they feel like their brains and their vaginas are synced up again. Once they had a treatment, whether it's hormone treatment or the more technical treatments, like radiofrequency or CO2 laser, it's as if there was a reconnection between the brain network and their vaginas. For this reason, perhaps, the frequency and intensity of orgasm improves for many. With these new technologies, women are experiencing dramatic improvements in their sexual and urinary health.

APPENDIX B

TEN-DAY SYMPTOM TRACKER

Record the date and the day of your menstrual cycle if you are still having cycles. List how well you slept the night prior and rate your energy level upon arising. What kind of mood have you been in most of the day? What symptoms are you experiencing: fatigue, irritability, headache, nasal congestion, constipation, difficulty concentrating? List all food and beverages consumed. On a scale of one to ten, what is your stress level and what is stressing you most today? And finally, what did you do to bring joy to your day? Or list what self-care looked like.

DATE	DAY OF CYCLE	SLEEP (# OF HOURS & QUALITY)	ENERGY (RATE ENERGY FROM 1-10)	MOOD

SYMPTOMS	FOOD DIARY	STRESSORS (RATE STRESS FROM 1-10)	JOY

APPENDIX C

MENOPAUSE MYTH JUMP-START

DECIDE THAT YOU ARE READY AND MOVE!

1. Take responsibility.

At the end of the day, it's your body and you are the most qualified to guide your healing. For too long, patients have put the doctor in the driver's seat. By now I hope you have come to appreciate the important role you play in managing your health. Do your homework. Research all medications you are taking.

2. Get your head right.

As objectively as possible, examine your symptoms, thoughts, and behaviors. Start with the Menopause Myth Ten-Day Symptom Tracker (Appendix B). Look for patterns and pay special attention to symptoms even twenty-four hours after eating.

3. Fix your food.

Start with a modified food elimination diet. Eliminate dairy, sugar, and gluten. Consider eliminating sugar only as a first step.

4. Find your guide.

If your current provider is not a good fit, see if they are willing to collaborate with other holistic practitioners. Find a provider that embraces Integrative / Functional medicine. Remember that it may take time to find a provider. Consider alumni directories of program in Integrative Medicine or practitioners of Functional Medicine.

Alumni of the University of Arizona's
Integrative Medicine Program:

https://integrativemedicine.arizona.edu/alumni_and_associates.html

Integrative Medicine - American Board of Physician Specialties:

https://www.abpsus.org/integrative-medicine

The Institute for Functional Medicine:

https://www.ifm.org/find-a-practitioner/

PERIMENOPAUSE/ MENOPAUSE LABORATORY CHECKLIST—KNOW YOUR NUMBERS

Irst off, create a system for you to keep up with all of your labs. I encourage every patient to take responsibility for monitoring their own labs. Don't assume that your provider has taken note of any lab trends. Patients who are present and aware of their labs and health status will facilitate their providers to be just that more engaged. Consider creating an Excel spreadsheet to keep up with the important labs. For example, if you're diagnosed with hypothyroidism you will want to keep up with the levels of all of the thyroid labs. If you are a borderline diabetic or officially diagnosed, you will want to keep up with all of the labs listed under blood sugar management. There is debate on whether hormones should be measured in saliva, urine, or blood. Salivary hormones may be more accurate for monitoring natural hormone levels. Patients on hormone replacement may benefit from twenty-four-hour analysis. There are several labs, including Genova (https://www.gdx.net/), Doctor's Data (https://www.doctorsdata.com), and ZRT (https://www.zrtlab.com).

Remember, levels may vary in terms of menstrual cycle. Interpretation can be tricky. I have not provided absolute ranges. Please see DrArianna.com for specific lab value details.

The following labs should be obtained as a baseline:

Thyroid Stimulating Hormone (TSH): This is the standard screening test to evaluate thyroid function. Providers practicing conventional medicine may only look at this hormone and also use a much higher cutoff than integrative/functional-medicine-practicing clinicians. Optimal values are debated, and knowing your baseline from youngest age may be helpful. TSH >/= 2.0 potentially represents diminished thyroid function.

Thyroid Peroxidase (TPO) and Thyroglobulin antibodies: These are antibodies that are diagnostic for Hashimoto's, an autoimmune condition that causes hypothyroidism. Many providers do not routinely evaluate these antibodies, even in patients diagnosed and treated for hypothyroidism. The presence of these antibodies indicate that the etiology of hypothyroidism is autoimmune. When Hashimoto's is active, there is also an increase in these antibodies.

Free T3: Free T3 is the active thyroid hormone that is *not* bound to proteins in the blood.

Testosterone (Free and Total): Testosterone is bound to SHBG. Most labs will provide both free and total levels. However, free levels are most accurately measured by determining total testosterone, sex hormone binding globulin, and albumin. Testosterone calculator takes into account SHBG and albumin. Download Testosterone Calculator App or input data into online calculators.

Hemoglobin A1C: Measures blood sugar over the past three months.

Follicular Stimulating Hormone (FSH): Typically measured on day three of the menstrual cycle to help determine a woman's fertility. It is also used as a screening test for menopause for the same reason. When there are many viable follicles, levels will be low. On the other end of the spectrum, the fewer functional follicles, the higher it will be. Follicle stimulating hormone will increase as menopause is approached. However, due to the fluctuations in estrogen FSH may remain low until estrogen levels consistently fall. FSH consistently over 40 U/L indicates menopausal levels.

Estradiol: There will be significant fluctuations of estradiol preceding menopause. Eventually levels begin to decline.

Progesterone: Depending on where you are in your cycle, progesterone levels will fluctuate.

hs-CRP: This is a biomarker for inflammation. It is also used as a screening tool for heart disease. Elevated levels are also seen in individuals with autoimmune conditions.

Vitamin D25 Hydroxy, D3 ng/ml: Considered a hormone and a vitamin that has an essential role in hormone balance.

Complete Blood Count

Lipids (Total Cholesterol, LDL, HDL, and Triglycerides)

Comprehensive Metabolic Panel: This panel includes electrolytes (sodium, potassium, CO_2, and chloride), kidney test (blood urea nitrogen and creatinine), glucose, calcium, albumin, total protein, bilirubin, and liver enzymes (alkaline phosphatase [ALP]), alanine amino transferase (ALT), and aspartate amino transferase (AST). It gives a general overview of metabolism, liver, and kidney function.

RESOURCES

Empowerment Tools

For a variety of high-quality, patient-recommended empowerment tools, toys, and products, check out the Tula Wellness and Aesthetics website: tulawellnessmd.com.

Pelvic Floor

For a full list of pelvic floor-strengthening products, visit Tula Wellness and Aesthetics webpage: tulawellnessmd.com.

Thyroid

For further reading on the controllable factors of thyroid disease, I recommend *Hashimoto's Thyroiditis: Lifestyle Interventions for Finding and Treating the Root Cause* by Izabella Wentz. Another excellent resource is *The Thyroid Connection: Why You Feel Tired, Brain-Fogged, and Overweight—and How to Get Your Life Back* by Amy Myers.

Self-Care

A great resource about daily rhythm is the book *The Miracle Morning,* by Hal Elrod.

Nutrition

An anti-inflammatory lifestyle begins at the food market. Stock your pantry with high-quality organic foods that will support your body's healthy functioning. One of the best resources to use while shopping for foods is Andrew Weil's Anti-Inflammatory Diet and Food Pyramid. His website (drweil.com) includes an interactive model that can be informative, and I also recommend that patients take a printed form with them for grocery shopping.

For thoughtful documentaries on the subject of food in our culture, see: *What the Health, Forks over Knives, Eating You Alive,* and *Supersize Me.*

ACKNOWLEDGMENTS

T o my parents who have supported me through it all—thank you is not enough. None of this was possible without your love and support.

My husband, Errol, whose patience and support have been the only way my dreams could be realized.

My son and daughter, Khalib and Maiya, for bringing me joy and while challenging me daily.

My staff at Tula Wellness who hold down the fort in my absence (Brandie, Andria, Yesica, Kim, Lynette, Eva, and Teresa). These ladies help make Tula the happiest place on earth for me and countless patients every day.

I have been so blessed with the love and support of my "tribe." Rayna Tibrey (sister from another mother), Maya Dillard Lidell, Jessica Gray, Leslie Williams, Laila Hishaw DDS, and Charlotte Jones-Burton, MD, Nicola Finley, MD, for your friendship and constant support.

Andy Weil, MD, and Richard Baxter for the support and mentoring. You have made more of a difference than you will ever know.

Christiane Northup, MD, author of *Women's Bodies, Women's Wisdom* and countless other publications that started the real conversations women need to be having among themselves. Thank you for being a REVOLUTIONIST. Reading your work was the beginning of my knowing that there was more to this than what I learned in medical school. Luann Brezendine, MD, author of *The Female Brain*, for your support and opening my eyes to complexities of hormones and brain chemistry.

Summer Flynn and Eland Mann, for taking my words and ideas and helping them come to life.

Zelema Harris and Cynthia Bond, for your support and confidence in my work.

Victoria Maizes, MD, for your daily leadership and support.

Kate Delaney, for being one of the most encouraging "badasses" I know.

There are so many more individuals that have made a powerful impact on my life. My patients, by far, have been the main inspiration for my personal growth and healing. There is not a day that goes by that I am not uniquely blessed to touch lives in awesome ways.

ABOUT THE
AUTHOR

D r. Arianna was born and raised in the South Bay area of Los Angeles, California. She received her undergraduate degree at Washington University in St. Louis and medical degree from Meharry Medical College in Nashville, Tennessee. She returned home to complete her ob-gyn residency at Martin Luther King Hospital and fellowship in maternal-fetal medicine at UCLA Medical Center. She is double-boarded in obstetrics/gynecology and maternal-fetal medicine.

Arianna Sholes-Douglas, MD, FACOG, has dedicated much of her career to helping women through all stages of life. After practicing high-risk pregnancy for over twenty years, she changed her focus from women of childbearing ages to women entering the second half of life. After graduating from the University of Arizona Integrative Medicine program founded by Dr. Andy Weil, she retired from maternal-fetal medicine and opened her practice, Tula Wellness and Aesthetics.

Dr. Arianna is the founder of and visionary behind Tula Wellness and Aesthetic Center, a unique medical practice incorporating an integrative approach to all care. "Tula" means "balance" in Sanskrit and her mission has always been clear: "uplift and empower women to live their best lives." She will celebrate thirty years providing care to women in 2019. Dr. Arianna lives in Tucson, Arizona, with her husband and two children.

OUR SERVICES

https://tulawellnessmd.com

Tula Wellness and Aesthetics is a full-service medical practice specializing in women and men's sexual health.

Services include:
- Medical Consultations
- Menopause Coaching
- Vaginal Rejuvenation
- Bioidentical Hormone Replacement
- IV Therapy
- Aesthetic Services
- Body Sculpting
- Laser Services
- Men's Sexual Health and Hormone Replacement

9 781599 328942